Welcome to ***"The Diabetic Cookbook and Meal Plan for College Students: 110+ Diabetic Recipes for College Success"!*** Navigating college life can be an exhilarating journey filled with new experiences, academic challenges, and personal growth. However, managing diabetes while juggling a busy schedule can add an extra layer of complexity to this exciting phase. This book is designed to be your comprehensive guide, offering practical solutions, delicious recipes, and strategic meal plans tailored specifically for college students living with diabetes.

Understanding the unique challenges faced by college students, we have curated over 110 diabetic-friendly recipes that are not only nutritious but also easy to prepare and budget-friendly. Whether you're living in a dorm with limited kitchen access, sharing an apartment with friends, or commuting from home, these recipes are crafted to fit seamlessly into your lifestyle. From quick breakfasts to fuel your morning classes, to hearty dinners that can be whipped up after a long day, this cookbook covers it all.

In addition to the recipes, we provide detailed meal plans that help you maintain balanced blood sugar levels while accommodating the fast-paced and often unpredictable nature of college life. Our meal plans are flexible, allowing you to mix and match recipes based on your schedule, taste preferences, and nutritional needs. We also include tips for grocery shopping on a budget, meal prepping in advance, and making smart food choices in dining halls and restaurants.

Living with diabetes doesn't mean you have to miss out on the joys of college life. With the right tools and strategies, you can enjoy a vibrant, fulfilling college experience while effectively managing your health. This cookbook aims to empower you with the knowledge and resources you need to make informed decisions, take control of your diet, and thrive both academically and personally.

So, whether you're a freshman just starting out, a seasoned upperclassman, or even a graduate student, this book is for you. Let's embark on this journey together and make your college years not only successful but also healthy and enjoyable. Here's to a balanced and delicious college life!

1. Scrambled eggs with vegetables

Ingredient:

- 3 large eggs
- 1 tbsp olive oil
- 1/2 cup diced bell pepper
- 1/2 cup diced onion
- 1 cup spinach or kale, chopped
- 1 tbsp low•fat milk (optional)
- Salt and pepper to taste

Instructions:

1. In a small bowl, beat the eggs with the milk (if using) and season with a pinch of salt and pepper.

2. Heat the olive oil in a non•stick skillet over medium heat.

3. Add the diced bell pepper and onion. Sauté for 2•3 minutes until softened.

4. Add the chopped spinach/kale and sauté for another 1•2 minutes until wilted.

5. Pour in the beaten eggs and use a spatula to gently stir and scramble the eggs, incorporating the vegetables.

6. Cook, stirring occasionally, until the eggs are fully cooked through, about 3•5 minutes.

7. Serve hot. Enjoy!

This recipe is high in protein from the eggs, and provides fiber, vitamins and minerals from the vegetables. The portion size is appropriate for a college student with diabetes. You can adjust the vegetable types based on your preferences. Enjoy!

2. Greek yogurt with berries and nuts

Ingredient:

• 1 cup plain Greek yogurt (full•fat or low•fat)
• 1/2 cup mixed berries (such as blueberries, raspberries, blackberries)
• 2 tbsp chopped walnuts or almonds

Instructions:

1. Scoop the Greek yogurt into a bowl.

2. Top the yogurt with the mixed berries.

3. Sprinkle the chopped nuts over the top.

That's it! This simple snack or light meal provides:

• Protein from the Greek yogurt to help keep you full

• Fiber, vitamins, and antioxidants from the berries

• Healthy fats and crunch from the nuts

The combination of protein, fiber, and healthy fats makes this a balanced and blood sugar•friendly option for a college student with diabetes. The natural sugars in the berries provide carbohydrates, while the nuts and yogurt help to slow the absorption of those sugars.

You can adjust the amounts of each ingredient to suit your preferences and hunger level. This is an easy, nutritious, and portable option that can be enjoyed anytime. Enjoy!

3. Omelette with spinach and feta cheese

Ingredient:

- 3 large eggs
- 1 tbsp olive oil
- 1 cup fresh spinach, chopped
- 2 tbsp crumbled feta cheese
- Salt and pepper to taste

Instructions:

1. Crack the eggs into a small bowl and beat them lightly with a fork. Season with a pinch of salt and pepper.

2. Heat the olive oil in a small non•stick skillet over medium heat.

3. Pour the beaten eggs into the skillet and let them sit for 30 seconds to a minute, until the bottom starts to set.

4. Use a spatula to gently push the cooked egg towards the center, tilting the pan to allow the uncooked egg to flow to the edges.

5. When the eggs are mostly set but still a bit runny on top, sprinkle the chopped spinach and crumbled feta cheese over half of the omelette.

6. Use the spatula to fold the other half of the omelette over the spinach and cheese.

7. Cook for another 1•2 minutes until the omelette is set.

8. Slide the omelette onto a plate and enjoy!

This omelette is packed with protein from the eggs, healthy fats from the olive oil and feta, and fiber and nutrients from the spinach. It's a balanced meal that will help keep blood sugar stable for a college student with diabetes. Adjust the fillings to your liking!

4. Chia seed pudding

Ingredient:

- 1/4 cup chia seeds
- 1 cup unsweetened almond milk (or milk of your choice)
- 1 tbsp maple syrup or honey (optional)
- 1/2 tsp vanilla extract
- 1/4 tsp ground cinnamon (optional)
- Fresh berries or sliced fruit for topping (optional)

Instructions:

1. In a medium bowl, whisk together the chia seeds, almond milk, maple syrup/honey (if using), vanilla, and cinnamon (if using) until well combined.

2. Cover the bowl and refrigerate for at least 2 hours, or overnight, stirring occasionally, until the chia seeds have thickened the mixture into a pudding·like consistency.

3. Divide the chia seed pudding into serving bowls or jars.

4. Top with fresh berries, sliced fruit, or any other desired toppings.

This chia seed pudding is a great option for a college student with diabetes for a few reasons:

- Chia seeds are high in fiber, protein, and healthy omega·3 fatty acids, which can help regulate blood sugar levels.

- The unsweetened almond milk provides creaminess without added sugars.

- The optional maple syrup or honey adds just a touch of natural sweetness.

- The fresh fruit toppings provide additional fiber, vitamins, and natural sugars.

You can easily adjust the recipe to your taste preferences and dietary needs. This makes for a satisfying, nutrient·dense breakfast or snack. Enjoy!

5. Cottage cheese with fruit

Ingredient:

• 1 cup low•fat or non•fat cottage cheese
• 1/2 cup mixed fresh fruit (such as berries, diced apple, diced peach, etc.)
• 1 tbsp chopped nuts or seeds (optional)
• Cinnamon or vanilla extract (optional)

Instructions:

1. Scoop the cottage cheese into a bowl.

2. Top the cottage cheese with the mixed fresh fruit.

3. If desired, sprinkle the chopped nuts or seeds over the top.

4. You can also add a dash of cinnamon or a splash of vanilla extract for extra flavor.

That's it! This simple snack or light meal provides:

• Protein from the cottage cheese to help keep you full

• Fiber, vitamins, and natural sweetness from the fresh fruit

• Healthy fats and crunch from the nuts/seeds (if using)

The combination of protein, fiber, and healthy fats makes this a balanced and blood sugar•friendly option for a college student with diabetes. The natural sugars in the fruit provide carbohydrates, while the cottage cheese helps to slow the absorption of those sugars.

You can adjust the amounts of each ingredient to suit your preferences and hunger level. This is an easy, nutritious, and portable option that can be enjoyed anytime. Enjoy!

6. Avocado toast on whole grain bread

Ingredient:
- 2 slices of whole grain or sprouted bread
- 1/2 ripe avocado, mashed
- 1 tbsp olive oil
- 1 tsp lemon juice
- Salt and pepper to taste
- Optional toppings: sliced tomatoes, crumbled feta, everything bagel seasoning, etc.

Instructions:
1. Toast the whole grain bread until lightly golden brown.

2. In a small bowl, mash the avocado with the olive oil, lemon juice, salt, and pepper until smooth.

3. Spread the mashed avocado evenly over the toasted bread slices.

4. Add any desired toppings.

5. Serve immediately.

This avocado toast is a great option for a college student with diabetes for a few reasons:

- Whole grain bread provides complex carbs, fiber, and nutrients compared to refined white bread.

- Avocado is high in healthy monounsaturated fats, which can help slow the absorption of carbs and keep blood sugar stable.

- The healthy fats, fiber, and moderate carbs from the bread and avocado make this a balanced meal or snack.

You can customize the toppings to your liking, such as adding sliced tomatoes, crumbled feta, or a sprinkle of everything bagel seasoning. The healthy fats, fiber, and moderate carbs make this a blood sugar•friendly option for a college student with diabetes. Enjoy!

7. Smoothies with low-sugar fruits like berries and avocado

Ingredient:

- 1/2 cup frozen mixed berries (such as blueberries, raspberries, blackberries)
- 1/2 avocado, peeled and pitted
- 1 cup unsweetened almond milk
- 1 tbsp chia seeds or ground flaxseeds
- 1 tsp honey or maple syrup (optional)
- Ice cubes (optional)

Instructions:

1. Add all the ingredients to a high•powered blender.

2. Blend on high speed until smooth and creamy, about 1 minute.

3. Taste and adjust sweetener if needed.

4. Pour into a glass and enjoy!

This smoothie is a great option for a college student with diabetes for a few reasons:

- Berries are low in sugar compared to many other fruits, providing fiber, vitamins, and antioxidants.

- Avocado adds healthy fats, fiber, and creaminess to the smoothie without spiking blood sugar.

- Chia seeds or flaxseeds provide additional fiber and healthy omega•3s.

- Unsweetened almond milk keeps the carb count low.

- The optional honey or maple syrup adds just a touch of natural sweetness if needed.

You can easily customize this smoothie by using different berry combinations or adding other low•sugar fruits like raspberries or blackberries. The healthy fats, fiber, and moderate carbs from the fruits make this a balanced and blood sugar•friendly option. Enjoy!

8. Low-carb pancakes made with almond flour

Ingredient:
• 1 cup almond flour
• 2 large eggs
• 1/4 cup unsweetened almond milk
• 1 tsp baking powder
• 1/2 tsp vanilla extract
• 1/4 tsp cinnamon (optional)
• Pinch of salt

Toppings (optional):
• Fresh berries
• Unsweetened shredded coconut
• Chopped nuts
• Sugar•free maple syrup

Instructions:
1. In a medium bowl, whisk together the almond flour, eggs, almond milk, baking powder, vanilla, cinnamon (if using), and salt until a smooth batter forms.

2. Heat a non•stick skillet or griddle over medium heat. Grease lightly with a small amount of butter or oil.

3. Scoop about 1/4 cup of the batter onto the hot surface, spreading it slightly to form a pancake shape.

4. Cook for 2•3 minutes per side, or until golden brown.

5. Repeat with the remaining batter, greasing the pan as needed.

6. Serve the low•carb pancakes warm, topped with your desired toppings.

These almond flour pancakes are a great option for a college student with diabetes because:

• Almond flour is low in carbs and high in healthy fats and protein, which helps stabilize blood sugar.
• The eggs and almond milk provide additional protein and healthy fats.
• The toppings like fresh berries, coconut, and nuts add fiber and nutrients without a lot of carbs.

9. Breakfast burrito with whole grain tortilla, eggs, and veggies

Ingredient:

- 1 whole grain or high•fiber tortilla
- 2 large eggs, scrambled
- 1/4 cup diced bell pepper
- 1/4 cup diced onion
- 1/4 cup spinach or kale, chopped
- 1 tbsp shredded cheddar cheese (optional)
- Salt and pepper to taste

Instructions:

1. In a non•stick skillet, sauté the diced bell pepper and onion over medium heat until softened, about 3•5 minutes.

2. Add the chopped spinach/kale and cook for 1•2 minutes until wilted.

3. In a separate bowl, scramble the eggs and season with a pinch of salt and pepper.

4. Add the scrambled eggs to the vegetable mixture and stir to combine.

5. Warm the whole grain tortilla according to package instructions.

6. Spoon the egg and vegetable mixture onto the center of the tortilla.

7. Top with shredded cheddar cheese if desired.

8. Fold the sides of the tortilla over the filling and roll up tightly to create a burrito.

This breakfast burrito is a great option for a college student with diabetes for a few reasons:

- The whole grain tortilla provides complex carbs, fiber, and nutrients compared to a refined flour tortilla.
- The eggs are a source of protein to help keep you full.
- The vegetables add fiber, vitamins, and minerals without a lot of carbs.
- The optional cheese provides healthy fats and a creamy texture.

The combination of protein, fiber, and complex carbs makes this a balanced and blood sugar•friendly breakfast. You can easily customize the fillings to your liking. Enjoy!

10. Overnight oats with unsweetened almond milk and nuts

Ingredient:
- 1/2 cup old·fashioned rolled oats
- 1/2 cup unsweetened almond milk
- 1 tbsp chia seeds
- 1 tbsp chopped walnuts or almonds
- 1 tsp cinnamon (optional)
- 1 tsp honey or maple syrup (optional)

Instructions:
1. In a mason jar or small bowl, combine the rolled oats, almond milk, chia seeds, and cinnamon (if using).

2. Stir to mix well.

3. Cover and refrigerate overnight or for at least 4 hours.

4. In the morning, stir in the chopped nuts and honey/maple syrup (if using).

5. Enjoy the overnight oats chilled or at room temperature.

This overnight oats recipe is a great option for a college student with diabetes for several reasons:

- Rolled oats are a complex carb that provides fiber to help regulate blood sugar levels.

- Unsweetened almond milk keeps the carb count low compared to dairy milk.

- Chia seeds add extra fiber, protein, and healthy omega·3s.

- Nuts provide healthy fats and a crunchy texture.

- The optional honey or maple syrup adds just a touch of natural sweetness if desired.

The combination of fiber, protein, and healthy fats in this recipe helps to slow the absorption of carbs and keep blood sugar stable. You can easily customize the toppings or adjust the sweetener to your taste preferences. This makes for a quick, portable, and nutritious breakfast or snack. Enjoy!

11. Grilled chicken salad with vinaigrette dressing

Ingredient:

For the Salad:
• 4 oz grilled chicken breast, sliced
• 2 cups mixed greens (such as spinach, arugula, romaine)
• 1/2 cup cherry tomatoes, halved
• 1/4 cup sliced cucumber
• 2 tbsp crumbled feta cheese (optional)

For the Vinaigrette Dressing:
• 2 tbsp olive oil
• 1 tbsp balsamic vinegar
• 1 tsp Dijon mustard
• 1 tsp honey (optional)
• Salt and pepper to taste

Instructions:

1. In a small bowl, whisk together all the dressing ingredients until emulsified. Set aside.

2. In a large salad bowl, combine the mixed greens, tomatoes, cucumber, and grilled chicken.

3. Drizzle the vinaigrette dressing over the salad and toss gently to coat.

4. Top with crumbled feta cheese if desired.

This grilled chicken salad is a great option for a college student with diabetes for a few reasons:

• Grilled chicken is a lean protein that won't spike blood sugar.
• The mixed greens and vegetables provide fiber, vitamins, and minerals without a lot of carbs.
• The vinaigrette dressing is made with healthy fats from olive oil, which can help slow the absorption of carbs.
• The optional feta cheese adds a creamy, salty element without too many carbs.

This salad is easy to prepare, portable, and provides a balanced meal with protein, fiber, and healthy fats to help manage blood sugar levels. Feel free to customize the salad ingredients to your liking. Enjoy!

12. Quinoa salad with vegetables and chickpeas

Ingredient:

- 1 cup cooked quinoa, cooled
- 1 (15 oz) can chickpeas, rinsed and drained
- 1 cup diced cucumber
- 1 cup cherry tomatoes, halved
- 1/2 cup diced bell pepper
- 1/4 cup diced red onion
- 2 tbsp chopped fresh parsley
- 2 tbsp olive oil
- 1 tbsp lemon juice
- 1 tsp Dijon mustard
- Salt and pepper to taste

Instructions:

1. In a large bowl, combine the cooked quinoa, chickpeas, cucumber, tomatoes, bell pepper, red onion, and parsley.

2. In a small bowl, whisk together the olive oil, lemon juice, Dijon mustard, salt, and pepper.

3. Pour the dressing over the quinoa salad and toss gently to coat.

4. Refrigerate for at least 30 minutes to allow the flavors to meld.

5. Serve chilled or at room temperature.

This quinoa salad is a great option for a college student with diabetes for several reasons:

- Quinoa is a whole grain that is high in fiber, protein, and complex carbs, which can help regulate blood sugar levels.
- Chickpeas provide additional protein and fiber.
- The vegetables add fiber, vitamins, and minerals without a lot of carbs.
- The olive oil and lemon juice dressing provides healthy fats to help slow the absorption of carbs.

You can easily adjust the vegetables based on your preferences or what's in season. This salad can be enjoyed as a main dish or a side. It's also portable and makes a great lunch option for a college student. Enjoy!

13. Baked salmon with steamed vegetables

Ingredient:

• 4 oz salmon fillet
• 1 tsp olive oil
• Salt and pepper to taste
• 1 cup broccoli florets
• 1 cup cauliflower florets
• 1/2 cup sliced zucchini
• 1 tbsp lemon juice
• 1 tsp dried dill (optional)

Instructions:

1. Preheat your oven to 400°F (200°C).

2. Place the salmon fillet on a baking sheet lined with parchment paper. Drizzle with olive oil and season with salt and pepper.

3. Bake the salmon for 12•15 minutes, or until it flakes easily with a fork.

4. While the salmon is baking, steam the broccoli, cauliflower, and zucchini until tender•crisp, about 5•7 minutes.

5. Drain the steamed vegetables and transfer them to a serving bowl. Drizzle with lemon juice and sprinkle with dried dill (if using). Serve the baked salmon alongside the steamed vegetables.

This baked salmon and steamed vegetable dish is an excellent option for a college student with diabetes for several reasons:

• Salmon is a lean protein that is high in heart•healthy omega•3 fatty acids.
• The steamed vegetables are low in carbs and high in fiber, vitamins, and minerals.
• The lemon juice and dill add flavor without any added sugars.
• The balanced combination of protein, healthy fats, and fiber•rich vegetables helps to regulate blood sugar levels.

This meal is easy to prepare, nutritious, and portable, making it a great choice for a college student with diabetes. Feel free to adjust the vegetable selection based on your preferences. Enjoy!

14. Turkey and avocado lettuce wraps

Ingredient:

- 4 oz sliced turkey breast
- 1/2 ripe avocado, sliced
- 2 tbsp plain Greek yogurt
- 1 tsp Dijon mustard
- 1 tsp lemon juice
- Salt and pepper to taste
- 4•6 large lettuce leaves (such as romaine or butter lettuce)

Instructions:

1. In a small bowl, mix together the Greek yogurt, Dijon mustard, and lemon juice. Season with a pinch of salt and pepper.

2. Lay the lettuce leaves flat on a plate or cutting board.

3. Divide the sliced turkey evenly among the lettuce leaves.

4. Top each lettuce wrap with a few slices of avocado.

5. Drizzle the yogurt•mustard dressing over the avocado.

6. Fold the lettuce leaves over the fillings to create the wraps.

These turkey and avocado lettuce wraps are a great option for a college student with diabetes for several reasons:

- Turkey is a lean protein that won't spike blood sugar.

- Avocado provides healthy fats to help slow the absorption of carbs.

- The lettuce leaves are low in carbs and high in fiber.

- The yogurt•mustard dressing adds flavor without added sugars.

This recipe is easy to make, portable, and provides a balanced meal with protein, healthy fats, and minimal carbs. It's a great option for a quick lunch or light dinner. Enjoy!

15. Stir-fried tofu with vegetables

Ingredient:

- 1 block (14 oz) extra•firm tofu, pressed and cubed
- 2 tbsp sesame oil
- 1 cup sliced mushrooms
- 1 cup broccoli florets
- 1 cup sliced bell pepper
- 1 cup shredded cabbage or spinach
- 2 cloves garlic, minced
- 2 tbsp low•sodium soy sauce or tamari
- 1 tsp rice vinegar
- 1 tsp sesame seeds (optional)
- Salt and pepper to taste

Instructions:

1. Heat the sesame oil in a large skillet or wok over medium•high heat.

2. Add the cubed tofu and stir•fry for 3•4 minutes until lightly browned on the edges.

3. Add the mushrooms, broccoli, bell pepper, and garlic. Stir•fry for 4•5 minutes until the vegetables are tender•crisp.

4. Add the shredded cabbage/spinach, soy sauce, and rice vinegar. Toss everything together and cook for 2•3 minutes more.

5. Remove from heat and season with salt and pepper to taste.

6. Sprinkle with sesame seeds if desired. Serve immediately over steamed brown rice or quinoa.

This stir•fried tofu dish is a great option for a college student with diabetes for a few reasons:

- Tofu is a lean protein that won't spike blood sugar.
- The vegetables provide fiber, vitamins, and minerals without a lot of carbs.
- The soy sauce and rice vinegar add flavor without added sugars.
- Serving it over a whole grain like brown rice or quinoa provides complex carbs.

The combination of protein, fiber, and complex carbs makes this a balanced and blood sugar•friendly meal. Feel free to adjust the vegetable mix to your preferences. Enjoy!

16. Zucchini noodles (zoodles) with marinara sauce

Ingredient:

- 2 medium zucchinis, spiralized or julienned into noodles
- 1 cup marinara sauce (look for a low•sugar variety)
- 2 tbsp grated Parmesan cheese (optional)
- Fresh basil leaves, chopped (optional)
- Salt and pepper to taste

Instructions:

1. Use a spiralizer, julienne peeler, or vegetable peeler to cut the zucchinis into long, thin noodle•like strips.

2. In a large skillet, heat the marinara sauce over medium heat until warmed through.

3. Add the zucchini noodles to the skillet and toss gently to coat with the sauce. Cook for 2•3 minutes, just until the zucchini is tender but still has a bit of bite.

4. Remove from heat and season with salt and pepper to taste. Serve the zucchini noodles with marinara sauce, topped with grated Parmesan cheese and fresh chopped basil, if desired.

This zucchini noodle dish is a great option for a college student with diabetes for a few reasons:

- Zucchini noodles are low in carbs and high in fiber, providing a healthier alternative to traditional pasta.

- The marinara sauce provides lycopene and other antioxidants without a lot of added sugars.

- The dish is easy to prepare and can be made in advance for a quick, portable meal.

- The combination of low•carb vegetables and a moderate amount of marinara sauce helps to keep blood sugar levels stable.

You can customize this recipe by adding grilled chicken, sautéed mushrooms, or other low•carb vegetable toppings. Enjoy this simple and nutritious zucchini noodle dish!

17. Cauliflower rice stir-fry

Ingredient:

- 1 head of cauliflower, riced (about 4 cups riced cauliflower)
- 1 tbsp olive oil
- 1 boneless, skinless chicken breast, diced
- 1 cup diced mixed vegetables (such as bell peppers, broccoli, carrots)
- 2 cloves garlic, minced
- 1 tbsp low•sodium soy sauce or tamari
- 1 tsp sesame oil
- Salt and pepper to taste
- Chopped green onions or cilantro for garnish (optional)

Instructions:

1. If using a whole head of cauliflower, pulse it in a food processor until it resembles rice•sized pieces. Measure out 4 cups of riced cauliflower.

2. In a large skillet or wok, heat the olive oil over medium•high heat.

3. Add the diced chicken and stir•fry for 3•4 minutes until cooked through.

4. Add the mixed vegetables and garlic. Stir•fry for 2•3 minutes until the vegetables are tender•crisp.

5. Stir in the riced cauliflower, soy sauce, and sesame oil. Cook for 3•4 minutes, stirring frequently, until the cauliflower is heated through.

6. Season with salt and pepper to taste.

7. Serve the cauliflower rice stir•fry hot, garnished with chopped green onions or cilantro if desired.

This cauliflower rice stir•fry is a great low•carb, high•protein option for a college student with diabetes. The cauliflower provides fiber and nutrients, while the chicken and vegetables make it a balanced, filling meal. Adjust the vegetable mix to your preferences. Enjoy!

18. Bean and vegetable chili

Ingredient:

- 1 tbsp olive oil
- 1 onion, diced
- 3 cloves garlic, minced
- 1 bell pepper, diced
- 1 zucchini, diced
- 1 can (15 oz) black beans, rinsed and drained
- 1 can (15 oz) kidney beans, rinsed and drained
- 1 can (15 oz) diced tomatoes
- 2 cups low•sodium vegetable broth
- 2 tbsp chili powder
- 1 tsp ground cumin
- 1 tsp dried oregano
- 1/4 tsp cayenne pepper (optional, for spice)
- Salt and black pepper to taste

Instructions:

1. In a large pot or Dutch oven, heat the olive oil over medium heat. Add the onion and sauté for 5 minutes until translucent.

2. Add the garlic, bell pepper, and zucchini. Sauté for another 5 minutes, stirring occasionally.

3. Stir in the black beans, kidney beans, diced tomatoes, vegetable broth, chili powder, cumin, oregano, and cayenne (if using). Season with salt and black pepper to taste.

4. Bring the chili to a simmer and let it cook for 20•25 minutes, stirring occasionally, until the vegetables are tender and the flavors have melded.

5. Serve the chili hot, garnished with any desired toppings such as diced avocado, shredded cheese, or chopped cilantro.

This chili is a great option for a college student with diabetes as it is high in fiber, protein, and vegetables, while being low in carbs and added sugars. The beans provide complex carbs and the vegetables add important nutrients. Adjust the spice level to your preference. Enjoy!

19. Grilled shrimp skewers with salad

Ingredient:

• 1 lb large shrimp, peeled and deveined
• 2 tbsp olive oil
• 1 tsp garlic powder
• 1 tsp paprika
• 1/2 tsp salt
• 1/4 tsp black pepper
• 4 cups mixed greens (spinach, arugula, etc.)
• 1 cup cherry tomatoes, halved
• 1/2 cucumber, sliced
• 2 tbsp balsamic vinegar
• 1 tbsp olive oil

Instructions:

1. Preheat grill or grill pan to medium•high heat.

2. In a bowl, toss the shrimp with 2 tbsp olive oil, garlic powder, paprika, salt, and pepper until evenly coated.

3. Thread the shrimp onto skewers, leaving a little space between each one.

4. Grill the shrimp skewers for 2•3 minutes per side, or until the shrimp are opaque and cooked through.

5. In a large salad bowl, combine the mixed greens, cherry tomatoes, and cucumber.

6. In a small bowl, whisk together the balsamic vinegar and 1 tbsp olive oil. Drizzle the dressing over the salad and toss to coat.

7. Serve the grilled shrimp skewers alongside the salad.

This recipe is diabetes•friendly as it is low in carbs, high in protein from the shrimp, and includes a nutrient•dense salad. The grilled shrimp and balsamic vinaigrette provide plenty of flavor without added sugars. Adjust portion sizes as needed to fit your individual dietary needs.

20. Stuffed bell peppers with ground turkey and quinoa

Ingredient:
• 4 medium bell peppers, halved and seeded
• 1 lb ground turkey
• 1 cup cooked quinoa
• 1 small onion, diced
• 2 cloves garlic, minced
• 1 tsp dried oregano
• 1/2 tsp ground cumin
• 1/4 tsp red pepper flakes (optional)
• 1/2 cup shredded low•fat mozzarella cheese
• Salt and black pepper to taste

Instructions:

1. Preheat oven to 375°F. Arrange the bell pepper halves in a baking dish.

2. In a skillet over medium heat, cook the ground turkey, onion, and garlic until the turkey is browned and the onion is translucent, about 5•7 minutes. Drain any excess fat.

3. Stir in the cooked quinoa, oregano, cumin, and red pepper flakes (if using). Season with salt and black pepper to taste.

4. Spoon the turkey•quinoa mixture evenly into the bell pepper halves. Top each one with a sprinkle of mozzarella cheese.

5. Bake for 20•25 minutes, until the peppers are tender and the cheese is melted.

6. Serve the stuffed bell peppers warm.

Tips for a college student with diabetes:
• The combination of protein•rich ground turkey, fiber•filled quinoa, and nutrient•dense bell peppers makes this a well•balanced, diabetes•friendly meal.
• Quinoa is a complex carb that won't spike blood sugar levels as quickly as simple carbs.
• Using low•fat cheese helps keep the fat and calorie content in check.
• Pair this with a side salad or steamed veggies for an even more nutrient•dense meal.
• Portion control is key • one stuffed pepper half makes a great serving size.

This easy, customizable recipe is perfect for a college student managing diabetes. Enjoy!

21. Cheese sticks or cubes

Ingredient:

- 8 oz block of low•fat cheddar or mozzarella cheese
- Optional seasonings: garlic powder, paprika, dried herbs

Instructions:

1. Cut the block of cheese into 1•inch cubes or long, thin sticks.

2. If desired, sprinkle the cheese pieces with any of the optional seasonings. Gently toss to coat.

3. Arrange the cheese sticks or cubes on a plate or in a container.

4. Serve immediately or refrigerate until ready to enjoy.

Tips for a college student with diabetes:
- Cheese is a great source of protein, which can help stabilize blood sugar levels.

- Look for low•fat or reduced•fat cheese varieties to keep the calorie and fat content in check.

- Pair the cheese with fresh vegetables like carrot or celery sticks for a balanced, diabetes•friendly snack.

- Portion control is key • stick to 1•2 oz of cheese per serving.

- The protein and fat in cheese can help slow the absorption of carbs, preventing blood sugar spikes.

This simple, customizable cheese snack is perfect for a college student managing diabetes. It's portable, satisfying, and nutritious.

22. Hummus with carrot and cucumber sticks

Ingredient:

- 1 (15 oz) can chickpeas, drained and rinsed
- 2 tbsp tahini
- 2 tbsp fresh lemon juice
- 1 garlic clove, minced
- 1/4 tsp ground cumin
- 1/4 tsp salt
- 2·3 tbsp water, as needed for blending
- 2 medium carrots, peeled and cut into sticks
- 1 English cucumber, cut into sticks

Instructions:

1. In a food processor or high·powered blender, combine the chickpeas, tahini, lemon juice, garlic, cumin, and salt. Blend until smooth, adding 2·3 tbsp of water as needed to reach your desired consistency.

2. Transfer the hummus to a serving bowl.

3. Arrange the carrot and cucumber sticks around the hummus.

4. Serve immediately or refrigerate until ready to enjoy.

Tips for a college student with diabetes:

- The fiber, protein, and healthy fats in the hummus and veggies make this a great diabetes·friendly snack.

- The complex carbs from the chickpeas and veggies won't spike blood sugar levels as quickly as simple carbs.

- Pair this with a lean protein like grilled chicken or hard·boiled eggs for a more substantial meal.

- Portion control is key · stick to 1/4 cup of hummus and 1 cup of veggies per serving.

This easy, nutritious snack is perfect for a busy college student managing diabetes. Enjoy!

23. Hard-boiled eggs

Ingredient:

- 2 slices whole grain or sourdough bread
- 1 ripe avocado, mashed
- 2 hard•boiled eggs, peeled and sliced
- 1 tbsp olive oil
- 1 tsp lemon juice
- Salt and pepper to taste
- Optional toppings: red pepper flakes, everything bagel seasoning, chopped fresh herbs

Instructions:

1. Bring a pot of water to a boil. Carefully add the eggs and cook for 12 minutes for hard•boiled. Drain, cool, and peel the eggs.

2. Slice or mash the avocado in a small bowl. Stir in the olive oil, lemon juice, and a pinch of salt and pepper.

3. Toast the bread slices until golden brown.

4. Spread the mashed avocado evenly over the toasted bread slices.

5. Top each slice with sliced hard•boiled egg.

6. Sprinkle with any desired toppings, such as red pepper flakes, everything bagel seasoning, or chopped fresh herbs.

7. Serve immediately.

Tips:
- Use ripe, creamy avocados for the best flavor and texture.
- Adjust the amount of lemon juice to your taste preference.
- For extra protein, you can also add a drizzle of olive oil or a sprinkle of hemp seeds.
- This makes a satisfying, nutrient•dense breakfast or snack.

Enjoy this simple, yet delicious avocado toast topped with the protein•rich addition of hard•boiled eggs!

24. Almonds or other nuts (in moderation)

Ingredient:
- 1 lb boneless, skinless chicken tenders
- 1 cup almond flour
- 1 tsp garlic powder
- 1 tsp paprika
- 1/2 tsp salt
- 1/4 tsp black pepper
- 2 eggs, beaten
- Olive oil or avocado oil for cooking

Instructions:

1. Preheat oven to 400°F and line a baking sheet with parchment paper.

2. In a shallow bowl, mix together the almond flour, garlic powder, paprika, salt, and pepper.

3. Dip the chicken tenders into the beaten eggs, then dredge them in the almond flour mixture, pressing to help it adhere.

4. In a large skillet, heat about 2 tablespoons of oil over medium•high heat.

5. Working in batches, add the coated chicken tenders to the hot oil and cook for 2•3 minutes per side until golden brown.

6. Transfer the seared chicken tenders to the prepared baking sheet.

7. Bake for 10•12 minutes, flipping halfway, until the chicken is cooked through and reaches an internal temperature of 165°F.

8. Serve the almond•crusted chicken tenders warm, with your favorite dipping sauce on the side.

Enjoy this healthier, low•carb take on classic chicken tenders! The almond flour creates a delicious crispy coating.

25. Edamame (steamed soybeans)

Ingredient:

- 1 cup shelled edamame, cooked and cooled
- 2 ripe avocados, pitted and mashed
- 1/4 cup diced red onion
- 2 tablespoons chopped cilantro
- 1 tablespoon lime juice
- 1 garlic clove, minced
- 1/2 teaspoon salt
- 1/4 teaspoon ground cumin
- Pinch of cayenne pepper (optional)

Instructions:

1. In a medium bowl, mash the avocados with a fork or potato masher until slightly chunky.

2. Add the cooked edamame, red onion, cilantro, lime juice, garlic, salt, cumin, and cayenne (if using). Stir to combine.

3. Taste and adjust seasonings as needed, adding more lime juice for acidity, salt for flavor, or cayenne for heat.

4. Serve the edamame guacamole immediately with tortilla chips, veggie sticks, or as a topping for tacos, burgers, or grilled meats.

Tips:
- Use fresh, ripe avocados for the best flavor and texture.

- Cooking the edamame ahead of time makes it easy to incorporate into the guacamole.

- For a creamier texture, you can blend the edamame with the avocado in a food processor.

- Adjust the amount of lime juice and seasonings to your personal taste preferences.

This edamame guacamole is a delicious, nutrient•dense twist on classic guacamole. The edamame adds extra protein, fiber, and a pop of green color. Enjoy it as a healthy dip or topping.

26. Apple slices with almond butter

Ingredient:
- 1 medium apple, cored and sliced into thin wedges
- 2 tablespoons natural almond butter

Instructions:
1. Wash and slice the apple into thin wedges or slices.
2. Spread about 1•2 teaspoons of almond butter onto each apple slice.

Nutrition Information (per serving):
- Calories: 150
- Total Carbs: 15g
- Fiber: 4g
- Net Carbs: 11g
- Protein: 5g
- Fat: 9g

This snack is a great option for a college student with diabetes. The apple provides fiber, vitamins, and natural sweetness, while the almond butter adds healthy fats and protein to help balance blood sugar levels. The combination of the fruit and nut butter makes for a satisfying and nutritious snack.

Remember to monitor your blood sugar when eating this, as the carbs from the apple can impact your levels. Adjust the portion size as needed to keep your blood sugar in a healthy range. Enjoy!

27. Rice cakes with avocado

Ingredient:

- 2 whole grain rice cakes
- 1/2 ripe avocado, mashed
- 1 tsp lemon juice
- Salt and pepper to taste

Instructions:

1. In a small bowl, mash the avocado with the lemon juice. Season with a pinch of salt and pepper.

2. Spread the mashed avocado evenly over the rice cakes.

Nutrition Information (per serving):
- Calories: 180
- Total Carbs: 20g
- Fiber: 5g
- Net Carbs: 15g
- Protein: 3g
- Fat: 10g

This snack is a great option for a college student with diabetes. The rice cakes provide complex carbs, while the avocado adds healthy fats, fiber, and a creamy texture. The combination helps to slow the absorption of the carbs and keep blood sugar levels more stable.

Remember to monitor your blood sugar when eating this, as the carbs from the rice cakes can impact your levels. Adjust the portion size as needed to keep your blood sugar in a healthy range. Enjoy!

28. Greek yogurt with a sprinkle of nuts/seeds

Ingredient:
• 1 cup plain Greek yogurt
• 1•2 tbsp mixed nuts and seeds (such as almonds, walnuts, pumpkin seeds, chia seeds)
• Optional: 1•2 tsp honey or maple syrup (for extra sweetness)

Instructions:
1. Scoop the Greek yogurt into a bowl.
2. Sprinkle the mixed nuts and seeds over the top of the yogurt.
3. If desired, drizzle a small amount of honey or maple syrup over the top.

Nutrition Information (per serving):
• Calories: 200
• Total Carbs: 12g
• Fiber: 3g
• Net Carbs: 9g
• Protein: 18g
• Fat: 10g

This snack is a great option for a college student with diabetes. The Greek yogurt provides protein and probiotics, while the nuts and seeds add healthy fats, fiber, and a satisfying crunch. The combination helps to keep blood sugar levels stable.

Remember to monitor your blood sugar when eating this, as the carbs from the yogurt and any added sweetener can impact your levels. Adjust the portion size as needed to keep your blood sugar in a healthy range. Enjoy!

29. Cottage cheese with cherry tomatoes

Ingredient:

- 1/2 cup low·fat or non·fat cottage cheese
- 1/2 cup cherry tomatoes, halved
- 1 tsp fresh chopped basil (optional)
- Salt and pepper to taste

Instructions:

1. Place the cottage cheese in a small bowl.

2. Top the cottage cheese with the halved cherry tomatoes.

3. Sprinkle the fresh chopped basil over the top, if using.

4. Season with a pinch of salt and pepper.

This snack provides a nice balance of protein, healthy fats, and fiber to help manage blood sugar levels. The cottage cheese is a good source of protein, while the cherry tomatoes provide vitamins, minerals, and antioxidants. The basil adds a fresh flavor and a little extra nutrition.

This is a quick, easy, and portable snack that a college student with diabetes could enjoy. The combination of the creamy cottage cheese and juicy tomatoes makes for a tasty and satisfying treat. Adjust the portion sizes as needed to fit your dietary needs.

30. Seaweed snacks

Ingredient:
• Sheets of dried seaweed (nori)
• Olive oil or sesame oil
• Salt, soy sauce, or other seasonings (optional)

Instructions:
1. Preheat oven to 300°F.

2. Cut the seaweed sheets into bite•sized pieces or strips.

3. Lightly brush or spray the seaweed with oil.

4. Season with salt, soy sauce, or other desired seasonings.

5. Arrange the seaweed pieces in a single layer on a baking sheet.

6. Bake for 5•10 minutes, until crispy. Watch closely to prevent burning. Allow to cool before serving.

Spicy Seaweed Snacks
Ingredients:
• Sheets of dried seaweed (nori)
• Sesame oil
• Gochugaru (Korean chili flakes) or cayenne pepper
• Soy sauce or salt

Instructions:
1. Cut the seaweed sheets into bite•sized pieces.

2. In a bowl, toss the seaweed pieces with a drizzle of sesame oil to lightly coat.

3. Sprinkle on the gochugaru or cayenne pepper and toss to evenly distribute.

4. Add a splash of soy sauce or a pinch of salt and toss again.

5. Spread the seasoned seaweed pieces in a single layer on a baking sheet.

6. Bake at 300°F for 5•10 minutes, until crispy. Allow to cool before serving.

31. Chicken and vegetable soup

Ingredient:

- 4 cups low•sodium chicken broth
- 1 boneless, skinless chicken breast, cubed
- 1 cup diced carrots
- 1 cup diced celery
- 1 cup diced zucchini
- 1/2 cup diced onion
- 2 cloves garlic, minced
- 1 tsp dried thyme
- 1 bay leaf
- Salt and pepper to taste

Instructions:

1. In a large pot, bring the chicken broth to a simmer over medium heat.

2. Add the cubed chicken, carrots, celery, zucchini, onion, and garlic. Season with the thyme, bay leaf, salt, and pepper.

3. Reduce heat to low and let the soup simmer for 20•25 minutes, or until the chicken is cooked through and the vegetables are tender.

4. Remove the bay leaf before serving.

This soup is a great option for a college student with diabetes for a few reasons:

- The lean chicken breast provides protein to help stabilize blood sugar levels.

- The vegetables are low in carbs and high in fiber, which helps slow the absorption of sugars.

- The low•sodium broth keeps the sodium content in check.

- It's a one•dish meal that's easy to prepare and pack for lunch.

You can adjust the vegetable mix to include your favorites. Spinach, kale, or other greens would also be great additions. Serve with a small whole grain roll or crackers for a complete and balanced meal.

32. Lentil soup

Ingredient:

- 1 cup dry brown or green lentils, rinsed
- 4 cups low•sodium vegetable or chicken broth
- 1 medium onion, diced
- 2 carrots, peeled and diced
- 2 celery stalks, diced
- 3 garlic cloves, minced
- 1 tsp ground cumin
- 1 tsp dried oregano
- Salt and pepper to taste
- Optional: 1 cup diced tomatoes (canned or fresh)

Instructions:

1. In a large pot, combine the lentils and broth. Bring to a boil over high heat.

2. Reduce heat to medium•low, cover and simmer for 15•20 minutes, until lentils are tender.

3. Add the onion, carrots, celery, garlic, cumin, oregano, and salt and pepper to taste. Simmer for an additional 10•15 minutes, until vegetables are tender.

4. If using, stir in the diced tomatoes and cook for 5 more minutes. Adjust seasoning as needed.

Nutrition Information (per serving):
- Calories: 250
- Total Carbs: 35g
- Fiber: 12g
- Net Carbs: 23g
- Protein: 15g
- Fat: 3g

This lentil soup is a great option for a college student with diabetes. Lentils are a complex carb that is high in fiber, which helps to slow the absorption of carbs and keep blood sugar levels stable. The vegetables and spices also add beneficial nutrients without a lot of extra carbs.

Remember to monitor your blood sugar when eating this, as the carbs from the lentils can impact your levels. Adjust the portion size as needed to keep your blood sugar in a healthy range. Enjoy!

33. Minestrone soup (with whole grain pasta)

Ingredient:

- 2 tbsp olive oil
- 1 onion, diced
- 3 carrots, peeled and diced
- 3 celery stalks, diced
- 3 garlic cloves, minced
- 1 (15 oz) can diced tomatoes
- 4 cups low•sodium vegetable or chicken broth
- 1 (15 oz) can kidney beans, drained and rinsed
- 1 cup whole grain elbow macaroni or small pasta
- 2 cups chopped kale or spinach
- 2 tsp dried Italian seasoning
- Salt and pepper to taste
- Grated Parmesan cheese (optional)

Instructions:

1. In a large pot, heat the olive oil over medium heat. Add the diced onion, carrots, and celery. Sauté for 5•7 minutes until softened.

2. Add the minced garlic and sauté for 1 minute until fragrant.

3. Pour in the diced tomatoes and broth. Stir in the kidney beans, whole grain pasta, kale/spinach, and Italian seasoning. Season with salt and pepper.

4. Bring the soup to a boil, then reduce heat and let simmer for 15•20 minutes, until the pasta is tender.

5. Ladle the minestrone soup into bowls and top with a sprinkle of grated Parmesan cheese, if desired.

This minestrone soup is an excellent choice for a college student with diabetes for a few reasons:

- The whole grain pasta provides complex carbs and fiber to help manage blood sugar.
- The beans, vegetables, and greens add important nutrients without a lot of carbs.
- It's a hearty, one•dish meal that's easy to make and pack for lunch.
- The simple ingredient list makes it budget•friendly for a college student.

34. Tomato basil soup

Ingredient:

- 2 tbsp olive oil
- 1 onion, diced
- 3 garlic cloves, minced
- 1 (28 oz) can crushed tomatoes
- 2 cups low•sodium chicken or vegetable broth
- 1 tsp dried basil
- 1/2 tsp dried oregano
- 1/4 tsp red pepper flakes (optional)
- Salt and pepper to taste
- 1/4 cup fresh basil leaves, chopped
- Grated Parmesan cheese (optional)

Instructions:

1. In a large pot, heat the olive oil over medium heat. Add the diced onion and sauté for 5•7 minutes until translucent.

2. Add the minced garlic and sauté for 1 minute until fragrant.

3. Pour in the crushed tomatoes and broth. Stir in the dried basil, oregano, and red pepper flakes (if using). Season with salt and pepper.

4. Bring the soup to a simmer and let it cook for 15•20 minutes, stirring occasionally, to allow the flavors to meld.

5. Remove from heat and stir in the chopped fresh basil. Ladle the soup into bowls and top with a sprinkle of grated Parmesan cheese, if desired.

This tomato basil soup is a great option for a college student for a few reasons:

- It's packed with vitamins, minerals, and antioxidants from the tomatoes and fresh basil.
- The simple ingredient list makes it easy to prepare on a budget.
- It's a comforting, one•dish meal that can be enjoyed on its own or paired with a salad or grilled cheese sandwich.

You can customize the recipe by adding other vegetables like carrots, celery, or spinach. For a creamier texture, you can also stir in a splash of heavy cream or half•and•half at the end. Enjoy this flavorful and nourishing tomato basil soup!

35. Broccoli cheddar soup (using low-fat cheese)

Ingredient:

- 2 tbsp olive oil
- 1 onion, diced
- 3 garlic cloves, minced
- 4 cups low•sodium chicken or vegetable broth
- 4 cups chopped broccoli florets
- 2 cups low•fat milk
- 2 tbsp cornstarch
- 1 cup shredded low•fat cheddar cheese
- Salt and pepper to taste

Instructions:

1. In a large pot, heat the olive oil over medium heat. Add the diced onion and sauté for 5•7 minutes until translucent.

2. Add the minced garlic and sauté for 1 minute until fragrant.

3. Pour in the broth and add the chopped broccoli florets. Bring the soup to a simmer and cook for 10•15 minutes, until the broccoli is tender.

4. In a small bowl, whisk together the milk and cornstarch until smooth. Slowly pour the milk mixture into the soup, stirring constantly, and let it simmer for 5 minutes to thicken.

5. Remove the pot from heat and stir in the shredded low•fat cheddar cheese until melted and well incorporated.

6. Season the soup with salt and pepper to taste. Ladle the broccoli cheddar soup into bowls and serve hot.

This broccoli cheddar soup is a great option for a college student with diabetes for a few reasons:

- Using low•fat cheese and milk reduces the overall fat and calorie content.
- The broccoli provides fiber, vitamins, and minerals without a lot of carbs.
- The cornstarch helps thicken the soup without the need for heavy cream.
- It's a comforting, one•dish meal that's easy to prepare.

You can customize the recipe by adding other vegetables like carrots or cauliflower. Serve with a small whole grain roll or a side salad for a complete and balanced meal. Enjoy this creamy and cheesy broccoli soup!

36. Beef and barley soup

Ingredient:

- 1 lb lean beef stew meat, cubed
- 1 tbsp olive oil
- 1 onion, diced
- 3 carrots, peeled and diced
- 3 celery stalks, diced
- 3 garlic cloves, minced
- 6 cups low•sodium beef broth
- 1 cup pearl barley
- 1 bay leaf
- 1 tsp dried thyme
- Salt and pepper to taste

Instructions:

1. In a large pot or Dutch oven, heat the olive oil over medium•high heat. Add the beef cubes and brown on all sides, about 5 minutes total. Remove beef and set aside.

2. Add the onion, carrots, celery, and garlic to the pot. Sauté for 5•7 minutes until vegetables start to soften.

3. Pour in the beef broth and add the browned beef, barley, bay leaf, and thyme. Season with salt and pepper.

4. Bring the soup to a boil, then reduce heat and let simmer for 45•60 minutes, until the beef is very tender and the barley is cooked through.

5. Remove the bay leaf before serving.

This beef and barley soup is an excellent choice for a college student with diabetes for a few reasons:

- The lean beef provides protein to help stabilize blood sugar.
- The barley is a whole grain that is high in fiber, which helps slow the absorption of carbs.
- The vegetables add important nutrients and fiber without a lot of carbs.
- It's a hearty, one•dish meal that's easy to make and pack for lunch.

You can adjust the vegetable mix to include your favorites. Spinach, kale, or other greens would also be great additions. Serve with a small whole grain roll or crackers for a complete and balanced meal.

37. Spinach and white bean soup

Ingredient:

- 1 tbsp olive oil
- 1 onion, diced
- 3 garlic cloves, minced
- 4 cups low•sodium chicken or vegetable broth
- 1 (15 oz) can white beans, drained and rinsed
- 2 cups fresh spinach, chopped
- 1 tsp dried thyme
- Salt and pepper to taste
- Grated Parmesan cheese (optional)

Instructions:

1. In a large pot, heat the olive oil over medium heat. Add the diced onion and sauté for 5 minutes until translucent.

2. Add the minced garlic and sauté for 1 minute until fragrant.

3. Pour in the broth and add the drained and rinsed white beans. Bring the soup to a simmer.

4. Stir in the chopped spinach and dried thyme. Season with salt and pepper to taste.

5. Let the soup simmer for 10•15 minutes, until the spinach is wilted and the beans are heated through.

6. Ladle the soup into bowls and top with a sprinkle of grated Parmesan cheese, if desired.

This spinach and white bean soup is an excellent choice for a college student with diabetes for a few reasons:

- The white beans provide fiber, protein, and complex carbs to help manage blood sugar.
- The spinach is packed with vitamins, minerals, and antioxidants.
- The simple broth•based soup is light and easy to digest.
- It's a one•dish meal that's easy to make and pack for lunch.

You can adjust the recipe by using different types of beans or greens. Kale, chard, or other hearty greens would also work well. Serve with a small whole grain roll or crackers for a complete and balanced meal.

38. Miso soup with tofu and seaweed

Ingredient:

- 4 cups low•sodium vegetable or chicken broth
- 2 tbsp white or yellow miso paste
- 1 block firm or extra•firm tofu, cubed
- 1 cup sliced shiitake mushrooms
- 1 cup chopped spinach or kale
- 2 tbsp dried wakame seaweed
- 2 green onions, sliced
- 1 tsp grated fresh ginger (optional)
- Soy sauce or tamari, to taste

Instructions:

1. In a medium saucepan, bring the broth to a simmer over medium heat.

2. In a small bowl, whisk together the miso paste with a few tablespoons of the hot broth until smooth. Pour the miso mixture back into the saucepan and stir to combine.

3. Add the cubed tofu, mushrooms, spinach/kale, wakame seaweed, green onions, and ginger (if using). Simmer for 5•7 minutes, until the vegetables are tender.

4. Taste and adjust seasoning as needed, adding a splash of soy sauce or tamari.

5. Ladle the miso soup into bowls and serve hot.

This miso soup is an excellent choice for a college student with diabetes for a few reasons:

- The tofu provides lean protein to help stabilize blood sugar.

- The seaweed and vegetables add important nutrients and fiber without a lot of carbs.

- Miso is a fermented food that may have benefits for gut health.

- It's a light, nourishing meal that's easy to prepare.

You can adjust the vegetable mix to include your favorites. Bok choy, carrots, or other greens would also be great additions. Serve with a small whole grain roll or brown rice for a more filling meal.

39. Cauliflower soup

Ingredient:

- 1 head of cauliflower, cut into florets (about 4 cups)
- 1 tbsp olive oil
- 1 onion, diced
- 3 garlic cloves, minced
- 4 cups low•sodium chicken or vegetable broth
- 1 cup unsweetened almond milk
- 2 tbsp grated Parmesan cheese
- 1 tsp dried thyme
- Salt and pepper to taste
- Chopped fresh parsley for garnish (optional)

Instructions:

1. In a large pot, heat the olive oil over medium heat. Add the diced onion and sauté for 5•7 minutes until translucent.

2. Add the minced garlic and sauté for 1 minute until fragrant.

3. Add the cauliflower florets and broth to the pot. Bring to a simmer and cook for 15•20 minutes, until the cauliflower is very tender.

4. Using an immersion blender, carefully blend the soup until smooth and creamy. Alternatively, you can transfer the soup to a regular blender in batches and blend until smooth.

5. Stir in the unsweetened almond milk, Parmesan cheese, and dried thyme. Season with salt and pepper to taste.

6. Reheat the soup if needed, then ladle it into bowls. Garnish with chopped fresh parsley, if desired.

This creamy cauliflower soup is an excellent choice for a college student with diabetes for a few reasons:

- Cauliflower is low in carbs but high in fiber, vitamins, and minerals.
- The almond milk and Parmesan cheese provide creaminess without a lot of fat or carbs.
- It's a comforting, one•dish meal that's easy to prepare and pack for lunch.
- The simple ingredient list makes it budget•friendly for a college student.

40. Tofu stir-fry with broccoli

Ingredient:

- 1 block (14 oz) extra•firm tofu, cubed
- 2 tbsp low•sodium soy sauce or tamari
- 1 tbsp rice vinegar
- 1 tsp sesame oil
- 1 tbsp olive oil
- 3 cloves garlic, minced
- 1 inch piece fresh ginger, grated
- 4 cups broccoli florets
- 1/2 cup low•sodium vegetable or chicken broth
- 2 tsp cornstarch
- Salt and pepper to taste
- Cooked brown rice, for serving

Instructions:

1. In a medium bowl, toss the cubed tofu with the soy sauce, rice vinegar, and sesame oil. Let marinate for 10•15 minutes.

2. Heat the olive oil in a large skillet or wok over medium•high heat. Add the marinated tofu and cook for 5•7 minutes, turning occasionally, until lightly browned on all sides. Remove tofu from the pan and set aside.

3. In the same pan, add the minced garlic and grated ginger. Sauté for 1 minute until fragrant.

4. Add the broccoli florets and vegetable/chicken broth to the pan. Cover and cook for 3•5 minutes, until the broccoli is tender•crisp.

5. In a small bowl, whisk together the cornstarch with 2 tbsp of water to create a slurry.

6. Add the cooked tofu back to the pan with the broccoli. Pour in the cornstarch slurry and stir to thicken the sauce, about 1•2 minutes.

7. Season the stir•fry with salt and pepper to taste. Serve the tofu and broccoli stir•fry over a bed of cooked brown rice.

You can customize the recipe by adding other vegetables like bell peppers, snap peas, or mushrooms. Enjoy this quick, healthy, and delicious stir•fry!

41. Lentil stew

Ingredient:

- 1 tbsp olive oil
- 1 onion, diced
- 3 garlic cloves, minced
- 2 carrots, peeled and diced
- 2 celery stalks, diced
- 1 cup dried brown or green lentils, rinsed
- 4 cups low•sodium vegetable or chicken broth
- 1 (14 oz) can diced tomatoes
- 2 tsp dried thyme
- 1 bay leaf
- Salt and pepper to taste
- Chopped fresh parsley for garnish (optional)

Instructions:

1. In a large pot or Dutch oven, heat the olive oil over medium heat. Add the diced onion and sauté for 5•7 minutes until translucent.

2. Add the minced garlic, diced carrots, and diced celery. Sauté for 2•3 minutes until fragrant.

3. Stir in the rinsed lentils, broth, diced tomatoes, thyme, and bay leaf. Season with salt and pepper.

4. Bring the stew to a boil, then reduce heat and let simmer for 25•30 minutes, until the lentils are tender.

5. Remove the bay leaf. Taste and adjust seasoning as needed.

6. Ladle the lentil stew into bowls and garnish with chopped fresh parsley, if desired.

7. Serve with a side of whole grain bread or over cooked brown rice.

You can customize the stew by adding other vegetables like spinach, kale, or bell peppers. For a creamier texture, you can also stir in a bit of low•fat Greek yogurt at the end. Enjoy this nourishing and diabetes•friendly lentil stew!

42. Chickpea curry

Ingredient:

- 1 tbsp olive oil
- 1 onion, diced
- 3 garlic cloves, minced
- 1 tbsp grated fresh ginger
- 1 tsp ground cumin
- 1 tsp ground coriander
- 1 tsp garam masala
- 1/2 tsp turmeric
- 1/4 tsp cayenne pepper (optional)
- 1 (15 oz) can chickpeas, drained and rinsed
- 1 (14 oz) can diced tomatoes
- 1 cup low•sodium vegetable or chicken broth
- 1 cup frozen peas
- 1/4 cup plain Greek yogurt
- Chopped cilantro for garnish
- Cooked brown rice, for serving

Instructions:

1. In a large skillet or pot, heat the olive oil over medium heat. Add the diced onion and sauté for 5•7 minutes until translucent.

2. Add the minced garlic and grated ginger. Sauté for 1 minute until fragrant.

3. Stir in the cumin, coriander, garam masala, turmeric, and cayenne (if using). Cook for 1 minute to toast the spices.

4. Add the drained and rinsed chickpeas, diced tomatoes, and broth. Bring the mixture to a simmer and cook for 10•15 minutes, until slightly thickened.

5. Stir in the frozen peas and cook for 2•3 minutes more, until the peas are heated through.

6. Remove the curry from heat and stir in the plain Greek yogurt. Serve the chickpea curry over cooked brown rice, garnished with chopped cilantro.

You can adjust the spice level to your preference. Serve with a side of roasted vegetables or a fresh salad for a complete and balanced meal. Enjoy this delicious and diabetes•friendly chickpea curry!

43. Caprese salad (tomato, mozzarella, basil)

Ingredient:

• 1 pint cherry or grape tomatoes, halved
• 8 oz fresh mozzarella cheese, cut into 1•inch cubes
• 1/4 cup fresh basil leaves, chopped
• 1 tbsp balsamic glaze or reduced•balsamic vinegar
• 1 tsp olive oil
• Salt and pepper to taste

Instructions:

1. In a medium bowl, gently toss together the halved tomatoes, mozzarella cubes, and chopped basil leaves.

2. Drizzle the salad with the balsamic glaze and olive oil. Toss lightly to coat.

3. Season with a pinch of salt and freshly ground black pepper.

4. Serve immediately or refrigerate until ready to serve.

This caprese salad is an excellent choice for a college student with diabetes for a few reasons:

• Tomatoes and basil are low in carbs but high in vitamins, minerals, and antioxidants.

• Fresh mozzarella provides protein and healthy fats without a lot of carbs.

• The balsamic glaze adds flavor without a lot of added sugar.

• It's a refreshing, no•cook dish that's easy to prepare and pack for lunch.

You can customize the salad by using different types of tomatoes, such as heirloom or cherry. You can also add a sprinkle of pine nuts or a drizzle of high•quality extra virgin olive oil for extra flavor and nutrition.

Serve this caprese salad on its own or with a small whole grain roll or crackers for a complete and balanced meal. Enjoy this delicious and diabetes•friendly summer salad!

44. Stuffed mushrooms with spinach and cheese

Ingredient:

- 12 large mushrooms, stems removed and finely chopped
- 1 tbsp olive oil
- 1/2 cup finely chopped onion
- 2 garlic cloves, minced
- 1 cup fresh spinach, chopped
- 2 oz low·fat cream cheese, softened
- 1/4 cup grated Parmesan cheese
- 1/4 tsp dried thyme
- Salt and pepper to taste
- 2 tbsp shredded low·fat mozzarella cheese

Instructions:

1. Preheat oven to 375°F. Lightly grease a baking sheet.

2. Remove the stems from the mushrooms and finely chop them.

3. In a skillet, heat the olive oil over medium heat. Add the chopped mushroom stems and onion. Sauté for 3·4 minutes until softened.

4. Add the minced garlic and sauté for 1 minute until fragrant.

5. Stir in the chopped spinach and cook for 2·3 minutes until wilted.

6. Remove the skillet from heat and let the spinach mixture cool slightly. Then stir in the softened cream cheese, Parmesan, and thyme. Season with salt and pepper.

7. Stuff the mushroom caps evenly with the spinach and cheese mixture.

8. Arrange the stuffed mushrooms on the prepared baking sheet. Sprinkle the tops with the shredded mozzarella cheese.

9. Bake for 12·15 minutes, until the mushrooms are tender and the cheese is melted. Serve the stuffed mushrooms warm.

You can customize the filling by adding other vegetables or herbs. Serve these stuffed mushrooms as a healthy appetizer or side dish. Enjoy!

45. Eggplant Parmesan (baked, not fried)

Ingredient:

- 1 medium eggplant, sliced into 1/4·inch thick rounds
- 1 cup whole wheat breadcrumbs
- 1/2 cup grated Parmesan cheese
- 1 tsp dried oregano
- 1/2 tsp garlic powder
- 1/4 tsp salt
- 1/4 tsp black pepper
- 1 egg, beaten
- 1 (24 oz) jar low·sugar marinara sauce
- 1 cup shredded part·skim mozzarella cheese

Instructions:

1. Preheat oven to 375°F. Line a baking sheet with parchment paper.

2. In a shallow bowl, combine the breadcrumbs, Parmesan, oregano, garlic powder, salt, and pepper.

3. Dip the eggplant slices into the beaten egg, then dredge them in the breadcrumb mixture, pressing to adhere.

4. Arrange the breaded eggplant slices in a single layer on the prepared baking sheet.

5. Bake for 20 minutes, flip the slices, then bake for another 15·20 minutes until golden brown.

6. Spread 1/2 cup of the marinara sauce in the bottom of a 9x13 inch baking dish.

7. Arrange the baked eggplant slices in a single layer over the sauce. Top with the remaining marinara sauce and the shredded mozzarella cheese.

8. Bake for an additional 15·20 minutes, until the cheese is melted and bubbly.

9. Let the eggplant parmesan cool for 5 minutes before serving.

You can serve the eggplant parmesan on its own or with a side salad for a complete and balanced meal. Enjoy this delicious and diabetes·friendly baked eggplant dish!

46. Veggie burger (low-carb version)

Ingredient:
- 1 (15 oz) can black beans, drained and rinsed
- 1 cup cooked quinoa
- 1/2 cup almond flour
- 1 egg
- 2 tbsp chopped fresh parsley
- 1 tsp ground cumin
- 1/2 tsp garlic powder
- 1/4 tsp salt
- 1/4 tsp black pepper
- Olive oil or avocado oil for cooking
- 4 large lettuce leaves (such as romaine or bibb)
- Desired toppings (e.g. sliced avocado, tomato, onion, mustard, etc.)

Instructions:

1. In a large bowl, mash the black beans with a fork or potato masher until slightly chunky.

2. Add the cooked quinoa, almond flour, egg, parsley, cumin, garlic powder, salt, and pepper. Mix well until fully combined.

3. Divide the mixture into 4 equal portions and shape them into patties, about 1/2 inch thick.

4. In a large skillet, heat a drizzle of olive oil or avocado oil over medium heat.

5. Cook the veggie patties for 4•5 minutes per side, until lightly browned and heated through.

6. Serve the veggie burgers on large lettuce leaves, topped with your desired toppings.

You can customize the veggie burger by adding other vegetables, herbs, or spices to the patty mixture. Serve with a side salad or roasted vegetables for a complete and balanced meal. Enjoy this delicious and diabetes•friendly veggie burger!

47. Spinach and ricotta stuffed shells

Ingredient:

• 12 whole grain jumbo pasta shells
• 1 (15 oz) container part•skim ricotta cheese
• 1 cup shredded part•skim mozzarella cheese, divided
• 1/4 cup grated Parmesan cheese
• 1 egg
• 2 cups fresh spinach, chopped
• 2 garlic cloves, minced
• 1/4 tsp dried oregano
• 1/4 tsp salt
• 1/8 tsp black pepper
• 1 (24 oz) jar low•sugar marinara sauce

Instructions:

1. Preheat oven to 375°F. Cook the whole grain pasta shells according to package instructions until al dente. Drain and set aside.

2. In a medium bowl, mix together the ricotta cheese, 1/2 cup of the mozzarella, Parmesan, egg, spinach, garlic, oregano, salt, and pepper until well combined.

3. Spread 1/2 cup of the marinara sauce in the bottom of a 9x13 inch baking dish.

4. Stuff each cooked pasta shell with a heaping tablespoon of the ricotta•spinach mixture and place in the prepared baking dish.

5. Pour the remaining marinara sauce over the stuffed shells. Top with the remaining 1/2 cup of mozzarella cheese.

6. Bake for 20•25 minutes, until the cheese is melted and bubbly.

7. Let the stuffed shells cool for 5 minutes before serving.

This spinach and ricotta stuffed shells recipe is a great option for a college student with diabetes for a few reasons:

• Whole grain pasta provides complex carbs and fiber to help manage blood sugar.
• The ricotta and spinach filling is high in protein and low in carbs.
• Using part•skim cheeses reduces the overall fat and calorie content.
• It's a comforting, one•dish meal that's easy to prepare and reheat.

48. Ratatouille

Ingredient:

- 1 medium eggplant, diced
- 1 medium zucchini, diced
- 1 medium yellow squash, diced
- 1 red bell pepper, diced
- 1 onion, diced
- 3 garlic cloves, minced
- 2 tbsp olive oil
- 1 (14 oz) can diced tomatoes
- 2 tsp dried thyme
- 1 tsp dried oregano
- Salt and pepper to taste
- Chopped fresh basil for garnish (optional)

Instructions:

1. In a large skillet or Dutch oven, heat the olive oil over medium heat. Add the diced eggplant, zucchini, yellow squash, bell pepper, and onion. Sauté for 8•10 minutes, stirring occasionally, until the vegetables are starting to soften.

2. Add the minced garlic and continue cooking for 1•2 minutes until fragrant.

3. Pour in the can of diced tomatoes along with the thyme, oregano, salt, and pepper. Stir to combine.

4. Reduce heat to low, cover the pot, and let the ratatouille simmer for 20•25 minutes, stirring occasionally, until the vegetables are very tender.

5. Taste and adjust seasoning as needed.

6. Serve the ratatouille warm, garnished with chopped fresh basil if desired. It can be served on its own or over cooked whole grain pasta or brown rice.

This ratatouille is an excellent choice for a college student with diabetes for a few reasons:

- The vegetables are low in carbs but high in fiber, vitamins, and antioxidants.
- It's a one•dish meal that's easy to prepare and pack for lunch.
- The simple ingredient list makes it budget•friendly for a college student.
- Serving it over whole grain pasta or brown rice adds complex carbs and more fiber.

49. Vegetarian lettuce wraps with tofu and vegetables

Ingredient:

- 1 block (14 oz) extra•firm tofu, drained and cubed
- 2 tbsp low•sodium soy sauce or tamari
- 1 tbsp rice vinegar
- 1 tsp sesame oil
- 1 tbsp olive oil
- 1 red bell pepper, diced
- 1 cup sliced mushrooms
- 2 cups shredded cabbage or coleslaw mix
- 2 green onions, sliced
- 1 tbsp grated fresh ginger
- 2 garlic cloves, minced
- 1/4 cup chopped fresh cilantro
- 12•16 large lettuce leaves (such as romaine or bibb)
- Lime wedges for serving

Instructions:

1. In a medium bowl, toss the cubed tofu with the soy sauce, rice vinegar, and sesame oil. Let marinate for 10•15 minutes.

2. Heat the olive oil in a large skillet or wok over medium•high heat. Add the marinated tofu and cook for 5•7 minutes, turning occasionally, until lightly browned on all sides. Remove tofu from the pan and set aside.

3. In the same pan, add the diced bell pepper, sliced mushrooms, shredded cabbage, sliced green onions, grated ginger, and minced garlic. Sauté for 3•5 minutes until the vegetables are tender•crisp.

4. Add the cooked tofu back to the pan and stir to combine. Remove from heat and stir in the chopped cilantro.

5. To serve, place a few spoonfuls of the tofu and vegetable mixture into the center of a lettuce leaf. Wrap the lettuce around the filling.

6. Serve the lettuce wraps with lime wedges on the side.

You can customize the recipe by using different vegetables or adding a drizzle of peanut sauce or sriracha for extra flavor. Enjoy these fresh and healthy vegetarian lettuce wraps!

50. Roasted vegetable quinoa bowl

Ingredient:

- 1 cup uncooked quinoa, rinsed
- 2 cups low•sodium vegetable or chicken broth
- 1 medium zucchini, diced
- 1 red bell pepper, diced
- 1 cup broccoli florets
- 1 cup cherry tomatoes, halved
- 1 tbsp olive oil
- 1 tsp dried oregano
- Salt and pepper to taste
- 2 tbsp crumbled feta cheese (optional)
- 2 tbsp chopped fresh parsley

Instructions:

1. Preheat oven to 400°F. Line a baking sheet with parchment paper.

2. In a medium saucepan, combine the rinsed quinoa and broth. Bring to a boil, then reduce heat to low, cover, and simmer for 15•20 minutes, until quinoa is cooked and liquid is absorbed. Fluff with a fork.

3. In a large bowl, toss the diced zucchini, bell pepper, broccoli florets, and cherry tomatoes with the olive oil, oregano, salt, and pepper.

4. Spread the seasoned vegetables in a single layer on the prepared baking sheet. Roast for 20•25 minutes, stirring halfway, until vegetables are tender and lightly browned.

5. In a large bowl, combine the cooked quinoa and roasted vegetables. Toss to mix.

6. Top the quinoa bowl with crumbled feta cheese (if using) and chopped fresh parsley. Serve warm or at room temperature.

This roasted vegetable quinoa bowl is an excellent choice for a college student with diabetes for a few reasons:

- Quinoa is a whole grain that provides complex carbs, fiber, and protein to help manage blood sugar.
- The roasted vegetables are low in carbs but high in vitamins, minerals, and antioxidants.
- The optional feta cheese adds a creamy, protein•rich topping.
- It's a hearty, one•dish meal that's easy to prepare and pack for lunch.

51. Grilled or baked fish tacos with whole grain tortillas

Ingredient:

- 1 lb white fish fillets (such as tilapia, cod, or halibut)
- 1 tbsp olive oil
- 1 tsp chili powder
- 1 tsp cumin
- Salt and pepper to taste
- 8•10 small whole grain tortillas
- 2 cups shredded cabbage or coleslaw mix
- 1 avocado, sliced
- 1/4 cup chopped cilantro
- 1/4 cup plain Greek yogurt
- 1 lime, cut into wedges

Instructions:

1. Preheat grill or oven to 400°F.

2. Brush the fish fillets with olive oil and season with chili powder, cumin, salt, and pepper.

3. If grilling, place the fish on a lightly oiled grill grate and cook for 4•5 minutes per side, until fish flakes easily with a fork.
If baking, place the fish on a parchment•lined baking sheet and bake for 12•15 minutes, until cooked through.

4. Flake the cooked fish into bite•sized pieces.

5. Warm the whole grain tortillas according to package instructions.

6. To assemble the tacos, place some of the flaked fish in the center of each tortilla. Top with shredded cabbage, avocado slices, chopped cilantro, and a dollop of Greek yogurt.

7. Serve the fish tacos with lime wedges on the side.

You can customize the recipe by using different types of fish or adding other toppings like diced tomatoes, red onion, or a sprinkle of low•fat cheese. Serve with a side salad or roasted vegetables for a complete and balanced meal. Enjoy these delicious and diabetes•friendly fish tacos!

52. Shrimp and vegetable stir-fry

Ingredient:

- 1 lb shrimp, peeled and deveined
- 2 tablespoons olive oil
- 1 red bell pepper, sliced
- 1 cup broccoli florets
- 1 cup snow peas or snap peas
- 1 cup sliced mushrooms
- 3 cloves garlic, minced
- 1 tablespoon grated fresh ginger
- 2 tablespoons low•sodium soy sauce
- 1 tablespoon rice vinegar
- 1 teaspoon sesame oil
- Salt and pepper to taste
- Chopped green onions for garnish (optional)

Instructions:

1. Heat the olive oil in a large skillet or wok over high heat.

2. Add the shrimp and stir•fry for 2•3 minutes until they start to turn pink. Remove the shrimp from the pan and set aside.

3. Add the bell pepper, broccoli, snow peas, and mushrooms to the hot pan. Stir•fry for 4•5 minutes until the vegetables are crisp•tender.

4. Add the garlic and ginger and cook for 1 minute, until fragrant.

5. Return the shrimp to the pan. Pour in the soy sauce, rice vinegar, and sesame oil. Toss everything together and cook for 2•3 minutes more, until the shrimp are cooked through.

6. Season with salt and pepper to taste.

7. Serve the shrimp and vegetable stir•fry immediately, garnished with chopped green onions if desired. Enjoy over steamed rice or cauliflower rice.

This stir•fry is a great healthy and balanced meal. The shrimp provides lean protein, while the vegetables add fiber, vitamins, and antioxidants. The soy sauce, vinegar, and sesame oil add tons of flavor without needing to use a lot of salt or sugar.

53. Tuna salad with avocado

Ingredient:

- 2 (5 oz) cans tuna, drained
- 1 avocado, diced
- 2 tablespoons mayonnaise
- 1 tablespoon lemon juice
- 1 tablespoon finely chopped red onion
- 1 tablespoon finely chopped celery
- Salt and pepper to taste

Instructions:

1. In a medium bowl, gently mix together the drained tuna, diced avocado, mayonnaise, lemon juice, red onion, and celery.

2. Season with salt and pepper to taste.

3. Serve the tuna salad on lettuce leaves, in a sandwich, or with crackers.

The avocado adds a creamy texture and healthy fats to the classic tuna salad. The lemon juice helps prevent the avocado from browning. This makes a delicious and nutritious lunch or snack.

54. Baked cod with lemon and herbs

Ingredient:

- 4 (6 oz) cod fillets
- 2 tablespoons olive oil
- 2 tablespoons freshly squeezed lemon juice
- 1 teaspoon dried parsley
- 1 teaspoon dried dill
- 1/2 teaspoon garlic powder
- 1/4 teaspoon paprika
- Salt and pepper to taste

Instructions:

1. Preheat the oven to 400°F. Lightly grease a baking dish or line with parchment paper.

2. Place the cod fillets in the prepared baking dish.

3. In a small bowl, whisk together the olive oil, lemon juice, parsley, dill, garlic powder, and paprika.

4. Drizzle the lemon•herb mixture over the cod fillets and use a spoon to gently coat the fish.

5. Season the cod with salt and pepper to taste.

6. Bake for 12•15 minutes, or until the cod is opaque and flakes easily with a fork.

7. Serve the baked cod immediately, garnished with extra lemon wedges if desired.

This recipe is diabetes•friendly as it is low in carbs, high in protein from the cod, and uses healthy fats from the olive oil. The lemon and herbs add lots of flavor without needing to use high•sodium seasonings. Pair it with a side salad or roasted vegetables for a complete, balanced meal.

55. Fish curry with coconut milk

Ingredient:

- 1 lb white fish fillets (such as cod, tilapia, or halibut), cut into 1•inch pieces
- 1 tablespoon olive oil
- 1 onion, diced
- 3 cloves garlic, minced
- 1 tablespoon grated fresh ginger
- 1 tablespoon curry powder
- 1 teaspoon ground cumin
- 1 teaspoon ground coriander
- 1 (13.5 oz) can full•fat coconut milk
- 1 cup low•sodium vegetable or chicken broth
- 1 tablespoon lime juice
- Salt and pepper to taste
- Chopped cilantro for garnish

Instructions:

1. In a large skillet or pot, heat the olive oil over medium heat. Add the onion and sauté for 3•4 minutes until translucent.

2. Add the garlic and ginger and cook for 1 minute, until fragrant.

3. Stir in the curry powder, cumin, and coriander. Cook for 1 minute to toast the spices.

4. Pour in the coconut milk and broth. Bring the mixture to a simmer.

5. Gently add the fish pieces to the curry. Simmer for 8•10 minutes, until the fish is cooked through and flakes easily.

6. Remove from heat and stir in the lime juice. Season with salt and pepper to taste.

7. Serve the fish curry over cauliflower rice or with a side of steamed vegetables. Garnish with chopped cilantro.

This curry is diabetes•friendly as it's low in carbs, high in healthy fats from the coconut milk, and a good source of lean protein from the fish. The spices add lots of flavor without needing to use high•sodium ingredients. Enjoy!

56. Seared scallops with salad

Ingredient:

Scallops:
• 1 lb sea scallops, patted dry
• 1 tablespoon olive oil
• Salt and pepper to taste

Salad:
• 5 oz mixed greens
• 1 cup cherry tomatoes, halved
• 1/2 cucumber, sliced
• 1/4 red onion, thinly sliced
• 2 tablespoons olive oil
• 1 tablespoon balsamic vinegar
• 1 teaspoon Dijon mustard
• Salt and pepper to taste

Instructions:

1. In a large skillet, heat the olive oil over high heat.

2. Pat the scallops very dry with paper towels and season with salt and pepper.

3. Sear the scallops in the hot pan for 2•3 minutes per side, until a nice golden•brown crust forms. Be careful not to overcrowd the pan. Work in batches if needed.

4. Remove the seared scallops from the pan and set aside.

5. In a large salad bowl, combine the mixed greens, cherry tomatoes, cucumber, and red onion.

6. In a small bowl, whisk together the olive oil, balsamic vinegar, and Dijon mustard. Season the dressing with salt and pepper.

7. Drizzle the dressing over the salad and toss to coat. Divide the salad between plates and top with the seared scallops.

This meal is perfect for a college student with diabetes. The scallops provide lean protein, while the salad is full of fiber, vitamins, and healthy fats from the olive oil and vinegar dressing. The portion sizes are also diabetes•friendly. Enjoy!

57. Ceviche with lime and cilantro

Ingredient:

- 1 lb white fish fillets (such as tilapia, halibut, or cod), cut into 1/2•inch cubes
- 1 cup fresh lime juice (about 8•10 limes)
- 1 red onion, thinly sliced
- 1 jalapeño, seeded and minced
- 1 cup chopped fresh cilantro
- 1 avocado, diced
- 1 tomato, diced
- Salt and pepper to taste
- Tortilla chips or lettuce leaves, for serving

Instructions:

1. In a large non•reactive bowl (glass or stainless steel), combine the cubed fish and lime juice. Cover and refrigerate for 30•60 minutes, stirring occasionally, until the fish is opaque and "cooked" through the acid in the lime juice.

2. Drain any excess lime juice from the fish. Add the sliced red onion, minced jalapeño, chopped cilantro, diced avocado, and diced tomato. Gently toss to combine.

3. Season the ceviche with salt and pepper to taste.

4. Serve the ceviche immediately, either scooped into lettuce leaves or with tortilla chips on the side.

This ceviche is a great option for a few reasons:

- It's a light, refreshing, and flavorful dish that's perfect for warm weather.
- The lime juice "cooks" the fish without any heat, making it a no•cook meal.
- It's packed with lean protein from the fish, healthy fats from the avocado, and lots of fresh vegetables.
- The ingredients are simple and affordable, making it a budget•friendly option for college students.

You can customize the ceviche by using different types of fish or adding other vegetables like cucumber, mango, or red bell pepper. The key is to use the freshest, highest•quality ingredients you can find.

Serve this ceviche as an appetizer or a light main course. It pairs well with tortilla chips, tostadas, or a simple green salad. Enjoy this bright and zesty ceviche!

58. Smoked salmon rolls with cucumber

Ingredient:

- 4 oz smoked salmon, thinly sliced
- 1 medium cucumber, cut into 1/4·inch thick slices
- 2 tbsp cream cheese, softened
- 1 tbsp chopped fresh dill
- 1 tsp lemon juice
- Salt and pepper to taste

Instructions:

1. In a small bowl, mix together the softened cream cheese, chopped dill, and lemon juice until well combined. Season with a pinch of salt and pepper.

2. Lay the cucumber slices on a flat surface. Spread a thin layer of the cream cheese mixture onto each slice.

3. Top each cucumber slice with a piece of smoked salmon, trimming the salmon to fit the cucumber if needed.

4. Carefully roll up the cucumber slice with the salmon inside to create a small roll.

5. Arrange the smoked salmon rolls on a serving platter or plate.

6. Refrigerate the rolls for at least 30 minutes before serving to allow the flavors to meld.

These smoked salmon rolls are an excellent choice for a college student with diabetes for a few reasons:

- Smoked salmon is a lean protein that is low in carbs and high in healthy omega·3 fatty acids.
- Cucumber is a low·carb, high·fiber vegetable that provides crunch and hydration.
- The cream cheese adds a creamy element without a lot of carbs.
- It's a quick, easy, and portable snack or appetizer that can be made ahead of time.

You can customize the rolls by using different types of smoked fish, adding a sprinkle of capers, or using a flavored cream cheese. Serve these salmon rolls as a healthy snack or light meal. Enjoy!

59. Fish kebabs with vegetables

Ingredient:

- 1 lb white fish fillets (such as tilapia, cod, or halibut), cut into 1•inch cubes
- 1 red bell pepper, cut into 1•inch pieces
- 1 zucchini, cut into 1•inch slices
- 1 red onion, cut into 1•inch pieces
- 2 tbsp olive oil
- 1 tsp lemon juice
- 1 tsp dried oregano
- 1/2 tsp garlic powder
- Salt and pepper to taste
- Wooden or metal skewers

Instructions:

1. If using wooden skewers, soak them in water for 30 minutes to prevent burning.

2. In a large bowl, combine the cubed fish, bell pepper, zucchini, and onion. Drizzle with the olive oil and lemon juice. Sprinkle with the oregano, garlic powder, salt, and pepper. Toss gently to coat.

3. Thread the fish and vegetable pieces onto the skewers, alternating the ingredients.

4. Preheat grill or grill pan to medium•high heat.

5. Grill the kebabs for 8•10 minutes, turning occasionally, until the fish is cooked through and the vegetables are tender.

6. Serve the fish and vegetable kebabs immediately.

These fish kebabs are an excellent choice for a college student with diabetes for a few reasons:

- The lean white fish provides a good source of protein without a lot of carbs.
- The vegetables add fiber, vitamins, and minerals while keeping the carb content low.
- Grilling the kebabs is a healthy cooking method that doesn't require added oils or fats.
- It's a complete, balanced meal that's easy to prepare and pack for lunch.

You can customize the kebabs by using different types of fish or vegetables. Serve the kebabs over a bed of leafy greens or with a side of roasted sweet potato for a more filling meal. Enjoy this delicious and diabetes•friendly fish and veggie dish!

60. Grilled sardines with a side salad

Ingredient:

For the Sardines:
• 8 fresh sardine fillets
• 1 tbsp olive oil
• 1 tsp lemon juice
• 1/2 tsp dried oregano
• Salt and pepper to taste

For the Salad:
• 4 cups mixed greens (such as spinach, arugula, and kale)
• 1 cup cherry tomatoes, halved
• 1/2 cucumber, sliced
• 2 tbsp crumbled feta cheese
• 1 tbsp olive oil
• 1 tbsp balsamic vinegar
• Salt and pepper to taste

Instructions:

1. Preheat grill or grill pan to medium•high heat.

2. In a shallow dish, toss the sardine fillets with the olive oil, lemon juice, oregano, salt, and pepper until evenly coated.

3. Grill the sardines for 2•3 minutes per side, until cooked through and lightly charred.

4. In a large bowl, combine the mixed greens, cherry tomatoes, cucumber, and feta cheese.

5. Drizzle the salad with the olive oil and balsamic vinegar. Season with salt and pepper.

6. Serve the grilled sardines alongside the side salad.

You can customize the salad by adding other vegetables, nuts, or seeds. Drizzle with a bit of olive oil and balsamic vinegar or lemon juice for dressing.

Sardines are an affordable and nutrient•dense protein option that college students can easily incorporate into their diets. Enjoy this delicious and diabetes•friendly grilled sardine and salad meal!

61. Grilled chicken breast with asparagus

Ingredient:

• 4 (6 oz) boneless, skinless chicken breasts
• 1 tablespoon olive oil
• 1 teaspoon garlic powder
• 1 teaspoon dried oregano
• Salt and pepper to taste
• 1 lb asparagus, trimmed
• 1 tablespoon lemon juice
• 1 tablespoon grated Parmesan cheese (optional)

Instructions:

1. Preheat grill or grill pan to medium•high heat.

2. Rub the chicken breasts all over with the olive oil and season with the garlic powder, oregano, salt, and pepper.

3. Grill the chicken for 5•7 minutes per side, until cooked through and no longer pink in the center. Transfer to a plate and let rest.

4. In the same grill or pan, add the asparagus spears. Grill for 5•7 minutes, turning occasionally, until tender•crisp.

5. Transfer the grilled asparagus to a serving plate. Drizzle with the lemon juice and sprinkle with the Parmesan cheese, if using.

6. Slice the grilled chicken breasts and arrange them next to the asparagus.

Serve the grilled chicken and asparagus immediately. This makes a complete, diabetes•friendly meal that is high in protein, low in carbs, and full of nutrients.

The chicken provides lean protein to help keep blood sugar stable, while the asparagus is packed with fiber, vitamins, and minerals. The simple seasoning and lemon juice add lots of flavor without needing to use high•sodium or sugary sauces.

This is an easy, healthy, and satisfying meal that would be great for a college student with diabetes. Enjoy!

62. Chicken stir-fry with snow peas

Ingredient:
- 1 lb boneless, skinless chicken breasts, cut into 1•inch pieces
- 2 tablespoons olive oil
- 2 cloves garlic, minced
- 1 tablespoon grated fresh ginger
- 1 cup snow peas, trimmed
- 1 red bell pepper, sliced
- 1 cup sliced mushrooms
- 2 tablespoons low•sodium soy sauce
- 1 tablespoon rice vinegar
- 1 teaspoon sesame oil
- Salt and pepper to taste
- Chopped green onions for garnish (optional)

Instructions:
1. Heat the olive oil in a large skillet or wok over high heat.

2. Add the chicken pieces and stir•fry for 4•5 minutes until lightly browned and cooked through. Remove the chicken from the pan and set aside.

3. In the same pan, add the minced garlic and grated ginger. Cook for 1 minute until fragrant.

4. Add the snow peas, bell pepper, and mushrooms. Stir•fry for 3•4 minutes until the vegetables are crisp•tender.

5. Return the cooked chicken to the pan. Pour in the soy sauce, rice vinegar, and sesame oil. Toss everything together and cook for 2•3 minutes more.

6. Season with salt and pepper to taste. Serve the chicken stir•fry immediately, garnished with chopped green onions if desired. Enjoy over cauliflower rice or steamed brown rice.

This chicken stir•fry is a great diabetes•friendly meal option for a college student. The lean protein from the chicken, fiber from the vegetables, and healthy fats from the oils make it a balanced and nutritious dish.

The soy sauce, vinegar, and sesame oil provide lots of flavor without needing to use a lot of salt or sugar. Feel free to swap in other veggies you enjoy, such as broccoli, snap peas, or bok choy.

63. Baked chicken thighs with rosemary

Ingredient:

- 8 bone•in, skin•on chicken thighs
- 2 tablespoons olive oil
- 2 tablespoons chopped fresh rosemary (or 2 teaspoons dried rosemary)
- 2 cloves garlic, minced
- 1 teaspoon paprika
- 1/2 teaspoon salt
- 1/4 teaspoon black pepper

Instructions:

1. Preheat your oven to 400°F. Line a baking sheet with parchment paper or foil.

2. In a large bowl, combine the chicken thighs, olive oil, rosemary, garlic, paprika, salt, and pepper. Toss to evenly coat the chicken.

3. Arrange the chicken thighs skin•side up on the prepared baking sheet, making sure they are not touching.

4. Bake for 35•40 minutes, until the chicken is cooked through and the skin is crispy. The internal temperature should reach 165°F.

5. Optional step: During the last 5 minutes of baking, turn the oven to broil to further crisp up the skin.

6. Remove the baked chicken thighs from the oven and let rest for 5 minutes before serving.

This baked chicken thigh recipe is perfect for a college student with diabetes. The chicken thighs provide juicy, flavorful protein, while the rosemary, garlic, and paprika add lots of taste without needing to use a lot of salt or sugar.

Serve the chicken with roasted vegetables, a side salad, or cauliflower rice for a complete, diabetes•friendly meal. The leftovers also make a great protein•packed snack or lunch.

64. Chicken and vegetable kebabs

Ingredient:
- 1 lb boneless, skinless chicken breasts, cut into 1•inch cubes
- 1 red bell pepper, cut into 1•inch pieces
- 1 zucchini, cut into 1•inch slices
- 1 red onion, cut into 1•inch pieces
- 8 oz mushrooms, halved
- 2 tablespoons olive oil
- 2 tablespoons lemon juice
- 1 teaspoon dried oregano
- 1/2 teaspoon garlic powder
- Salt and pepper to taste
- Wooden or metal skewers

Instructions:
1. In a large bowl, combine the chicken, bell pepper, zucchini, onion, and mushrooms.

2. In a small bowl, whisk together the olive oil, lemon juice, oregano, and garlic powder. Pour the marinade over the chicken and vegetables and toss to coat.

3. Cover the bowl and refrigerate for 30 minutes to 1 hour, allowing the flavors to meld.

4. Preheat your grill or grill pan to medium•high heat.

5. Thread the marinated chicken and vegetables onto the skewers, alternating the ingredients.

6. Grill the kebabs for 12•15 minutes, turning occasionally, until the chicken is cooked through and the vegetables are tender.

7. Serve the chicken and vegetable kebabs immediately. Enjoy over a bed of cauliflower rice or with a side salad.

These kebabs are a great diabetes•friendly meal option for a college student. The lean chicken provides protein, while the vegetables add fiber, vitamins, and minerals. The marinade adds flavor without needing to use a lot of salt or sugar.

You can customize the vegetables based on your preferences or what's in season. Zucchini, bell peppers, onions, and mushrooms work well, but you could also use cherry tomatoes, eggplant, or asparagus.

65. Lemon garlic chicken with broccoli

Ingredient:

- 1 lb boneless, skinless chicken breasts, cut into 1·inch pieces
- 2 tablespoons olive oil
- 3 cloves garlic, minced
- 1 tablespoon lemon zest
- 2 tablespoons lemon juice
- 1 teaspoon dried oregano
- 1/4 teaspoon red pepper flakes (optional)
- Salt and pepper to taste
- 4 cups broccoli florets

Instructions:

1. In a large skillet, heat the olive oil over medium·high heat.

2. Add the chicken pieces and season with salt and pepper. Cook for 3·4 minutes per side, until lightly browned. Remove the chicken from the pan and set aside.

3. In the same pan, add the minced garlic and cook for 1 minute, until fragrant.

4. Stir in the lemon zest, lemon juice, oregano, and red pepper flakes (if using). Cook for 1 minute.

5. Add the broccoli florets to the pan and toss to coat in the lemon·garlic mixture. Cover and cook for 4·5 minutes, until the broccoli is tender·crisp.

6. Return the cooked chicken to the pan and toss everything together. Cook for 2·3 minutes more, until the chicken is cooked through.

7. Serve the lemon garlic chicken and broccoli immediately. Enjoy over rice, quinoa, or with a side salad.

This dish is packed with lean protein from the chicken, fiber and vitamins from the broccoli, and bright lemon flavor. The garlic, oregano, and optional red pepper flakes add lots of delicious seasoning. It's a quick and healthy weeknight meal.

66. Chicken lettuce wraps

Ingredient:

- 1 lb ground chicken or chicken breast, finely chopped
- 1 tablespoon olive oil
- 1 onion, diced
- 3 cloves garlic, minced
- 1 tablespoon grated fresh ginger
- 2 tablespoons low•sodium soy sauce
- 1 tablespoon rice vinegar
- 1 teaspoon sesame oil
- 1/4 teaspoon red pepper flakes (optional)
- Salt and pepper to taste
- 1 head of romaine or butter lettuce, leaves separated

Toppings (optional):
- Shredded carrots
- Sliced cucumber
- Chopped green onions
- Chopped cilantro
- Crushed peanuts or cashews

Instructions:

1. In a large skillet, heat the olive oil over medium•high heat. Add the ground chicken (or chopped chicken breast) and cook for 5•7 minutes, breaking it up with a wooden spoon, until no longer pink.

2. Add the diced onion and cook for 3•4 minutes until translucent.

3. Stir in the minced garlic and grated ginger. Cook for 1 minute until fragrant.

4. Pour in the soy sauce, rice vinegar, and sesame oil. Toss to coat the chicken mixture.

5. If using, stir in the red pepper flakes. Season with salt and pepper to taste.

6. To serve, place a few spoonfuls of the chicken mixture into the center of a lettuce leaf. Top with any desired toppings. Fold the lettuce leaf over the filling and enjoy.

These chicken lettuce wraps are a great diabetes•friendly meal option. The lean chicken provides protein, while the lettuce leaves keep the carbs low. The Asian•inspired flavors from the soy sauce, ginger, and sesame oil add lots of taste without needing to use a lot of sugar or salt

67. Chicken curry with cauliflower rice

Ingredient:

Chicken Curry:

• 1 lb boneless, skinless chicken breasts, cut into 1•inch pieces
• 2 tablespoons olive oil
• 1 onion, diced
• 3 cloves garlic, minced
• 1 tablespoon grated fresh ginger
• 2 tablespoons curry powder
• 1 teaspoon ground cumin
• 1 teaspoon ground coriander
• 1 (13.5 oz) can full•fat coconut milk
• 1 cup low•sodium chicken broth
• 1 tablespoon lime juice
• Salt and pepper to taste
• Chopped cilantro for garnish

Cauliflower Rice:

• 1 head of cauliflower, riced (about 4 cups)
• 1 tablespoon olive oil
• Salt and pepper to taste

Instructions:

1. In a large skillet or pot, heat the 2 tablespoons of olive oil over medium heat. Add the chicken and cook for 3•4 minutes until lightly browned. Remove the chicken from the pan and set aside.

2. In the same pan, add the diced onion and sauté for 5 minutes until translucent.

3. Add the garlic and ginger and cook for 1 minute until fragrant.

4. Stir in the curry powder, cumin, and coriander. Cook for 1 minute to toast the spices.

5. Pour in the coconut milk and chicken broth. Bring the mixture to a simmer.

6. Add the cooked chicken back to the pan and let the curry simmer for 10•15 minutes, until the chicken is cooked through.

7. Remove from heat and stir in the lime juice. Season with salt and pepper to taste.

8. Meanwhile, make the cauliflower rice. In a large skillet, heat 1 tablespoon of olive oil over medium heat. Add the riced cauliflower and sauté for 5•7 minutes, until tender. Season with salt and pepper. Serve the chicken curry over the cauliflower rice, garnished with chopped cilantro.

68. Chicken and spinach stuffed sweet potatoes

Ingredient:

- 4 medium sweet potatoes
- 1 lb boneless, skinless chicken breasts, cooked and shredded
- 2 cups fresh spinach, chopped
- 1/2 cup plain Greek yogurt
- 2 tablespoons grated Parmesan cheese
- 1 clove garlic, minced
- 1/4 teaspoon dried thyme
- Salt and pepper to taste

Instructions:

1. Preheat your oven to 400°F. Pierce the sweet potatoes several times with a fork.

2. Bake the sweet potatoes for 45•60 minutes, until fork•tender. Allow them to cool slightly.

3. Cut the sweet potatoes in half lengthwise. Scoop out the flesh into a medium bowl, leaving a thin layer of sweet potato in the skins.

4. In the bowl with the sweet potato flesh, mix together the shredded chicken, chopped spinach, Greek yogurt, Parmesan cheese, garlic, and thyme. Season with salt and pepper to taste.

5. Spoon the chicken and spinach mixture back into the sweet potato skins, dividing it evenly.

6. Place the stuffed sweet potato halves on a baking sheet and return them to the oven. Bake for an additional 10•15 minutes, until heated through.

7. Serve the chicken and spinach stuffed sweet potatoes immediately.

This dish is a great diabetes•friendly meal for a college student. The sweet potatoes are high in fiber, vitamins, and complex carbs, while the chicken provides lean protein. The spinach and Greek yogurt add extra nutrients and creaminess.

The portion size is appropriate for someone with diabetes, and the recipe doesn't require any added sugars or high•sodium ingredients. It's a simple, nutritious, and satisfying meal.

69. Teriyaki chicken skewers

Ingredient:

- 1 lb boneless, skinless chicken breasts, cut into 1•inch cubes
- 1/4 cup low•sodium soy sauce
- 2 tablespoons rice vinegar
- 1 tablespoon honey
- 1 teaspoon sesame oil
- 2 cloves garlic, minced
- 1 teaspoon grated fresh ginger
- 1/4 teaspoon red pepper flakes (optional)
- Wooden or metal skewers

Instructions:

1. In a medium bowl, whisk together the soy sauce, rice vinegar, honey, sesame oil, garlic, ginger, and red pepper flakes (if using).

2. Add the cubed chicken to the marinade and toss to coat. Cover and refrigerate for 30 minutes to 1 hour.

3. Preheat your grill or grill pan to medium•high heat.

4. Thread the marinated chicken cubes onto the skewers, leaving a little space between each piece.

5. Grill the chicken skewers for 8•10 minutes, turning occasionally, until the chicken is cooked through and no longer pink in the center.

6. Serve the teriyaki chicken skewers immediately. Enjoy them on their own or with a side of steamed broccoli or a fresh salad.

This teriyaki chicken skewer recipe is a great diabetes•friendly meal for a college student. The lean chicken provides protein, while the marinade adds tons of flavor without needing to use a lot of sugar or sodium.

The portion size is appropriate for someone with diabetes, and the dish is easy to prepare and transport, making it a convenient option for a busy college student.

You can customize the recipe by adding other vegetables to the skewers, such as bell peppers, onions, or mushrooms. Serve the chicken skewers over cauliflower rice or with a side of roasted sweet potato for a complete, balanced meal

70. Chicken fajita bowl (without rice)

Ingredient:

• 1 lb boneless, skinless chicken breasts, sliced into 1/2•inch strips
• 2 tablespoons olive oil
• 1 tablespoon chili powder
• 1 teaspoon cumin
• 1 teaspoon garlic powder
• 1/2 teaspoon smoked paprika
• Salt and pepper to taste
• 1 red bell pepper, sliced
• 1 green bell pepper, sliced
• 1 onion, sliced
• 1 avocado, diced
• 1/4 cup shredded cheddar cheese
• 2 tablespoons fresh cilantro, chopped
• Lime wedges for serving

Instructions:

1. Preheat your oven to 400°F. Line a baking sheet with parchment paper.

2. In a large bowl, toss the chicken strips with 1 tablespoon of the olive oil, chili powder, cumin, garlic powder, smoked paprika, salt, and pepper.

3. Spread the seasoned chicken in a single layer on the prepared baking sheet. Bake for 15•18 minutes, until the chicken is cooked through.

4. In a large skillet, heat the remaining 1 tablespoon of olive oil over medium•high heat. Add the sliced bell peppers and onion. Sauté for 5•7 minutes, until the vegetables are tender•crisp.

5. Divide the sautéed vegetables between 4 bowls. Top each bowl with the baked chicken, diced avocado, shredded cheddar cheese, and chopped cilantro.

6. Serve the chicken fajita bowls with lime wedges on the side.

This chicken fajita bowl is a great diabetes•friendly meal for a college student. It's high in protein from the chicken, packed with fiber and nutrients from the vegetables, and has healthy fats from the avocado. By skipping the rice, you keep the carb count low.

71. Beef and broccoli stir-fry

Ingredient:

- 1 lb flank steak, thinly sliced against the grain
- 2 tablespoons low•sodium soy sauce
- 1 tablespoon rice vinegar
- 1 teaspoon sesame oil
- 2 tablespoons olive oil, divided
- 3 cloves garlic, minced
- 1 tablespoon grated fresh ginger
- 4 cups broccoli florets
- 1/2 cup low•sodium beef or chicken broth
- 1 teaspoon cornstarch
- Salt and pepper to taste
- Chopped green onions for garnish (optional)

Instructions:

1. In a medium bowl, combine the sliced flank steak, soy sauce, rice vinegar, and sesame oil. Toss to coat the beef and let marinate for 15 minutes.

2. Heat 1 tablespoon of the olive oil in a large skillet or wok over high heat.

3. Add the marinated beef to the hot pan and stir•fry for 2•3 minutes until lightly browned. Remove the beef from the pan and set aside.

4. Add the remaining 1 tablespoon of olive oil to the pan. Stir in the minced garlic and grated ginger. Cook for 1 minute until fragrant.

5. Add the broccoli florets to the pan and stir•fry for 3•4 minutes.

6. In a small bowl, whisk together the beef broth and cornstarch. Pour this mixture into the pan with the broccoli.

7. Bring the sauce to a simmer and cook for 2•3 minutes, until thickened slightly.

8. Return the cooked beef to the pan and toss everything together. Cook for 1•2 minutes more, until the beef is heated through.

9. Season the beef and broccoli stir•fry with salt and pepper to taste. Serve immediately, garnished with chopped green onions if desired. Enjoy over cauliflower rice or zucchini noodles.

72. Grilled steak salad

Ingredient:

• 8 oz flank steak or sirloin steak
• 1 tablespoon olive oil
• Salt and pepper to taste
• 5 oz mixed greens
• 1 cup cherry tomatoes, halved
• 1/2 cucumber, sliced
• 1/4 red onion, thinly sliced
• 2 tablespoons crumbled feta cheese
• 2 tablespoons balsamic vinaigrette

Instructions:

1. Preheat grill or grill pan to medium•high heat.

2. Rub the steak with the olive oil and season generously with salt and pepper.

3. Grill the steak for 3•5 minutes per side, depending on thickness, until it reaches your desired doneness. Transfer to a cutting board and let rest for 5 minutes.

4. Slice the steak against the grain into thin strips.

5. In a large salad bowl, combine the mixed greens, cherry tomatoes, cucumber, and red onion.

6. Top the salad with the grilled steak strips and crumbled feta cheese.

7. Drizzle the balsamic vinaigrette over the top and toss gently to coat.

This grilled steak salad is an excellent diabetes•friendly meal. The lean steak provides protein, while the greens, tomatoes, and cucumber give you fiber, vitamins, and minerals. The balsamic vinaigrette adds flavor without a lot of added sugar. The portion size is also appropriate for someone with diabetes.

You can customize the salad by adding other veggies you enjoy, such as bell peppers or avocado. This makes a satisfying and nutritious lunch or dinner.

73. Pork tenderloin with roasted vegetables

Ingredient:

• 1 lb pork tenderloin
• 2 tablespoons olive oil, divided
• 1 teaspoon garlic powder
• 1 teaspoon dried thyme
• Salt and pepper to taste
• 1 lb Brussels sprouts, trimmed and halved
• 2 carrots, peeled and cut into 1•inch pieces
• 1 red onion, cut into 1•inch wedges
• 1 zucchini, cut into 1•inch pieces

Instructions:

1. Preheat your oven to 400°F. Line a large baking sheet with parchment paper.

2. In a small bowl, combine 1 tablespoon of the olive oil, garlic powder, thyme, salt, and pepper. Rub this seasoning mixture all over the pork tenderloin.

3. Place the pork tenderloin on one side of the prepared baking sheet.

4. In a large bowl, toss the Brussels sprouts, carrots, onion, and zucchini with the remaining 1 tablespoon of olive oil. Season with salt and pepper.

5. Spread the seasoned vegetables in a single layer on the other side of the baking sheet, next to the pork.

6. Roast the pork and vegetables for 25•30 minutes, until the pork reaches an internal temperature of 145°F and the vegetables are tender.

7. Remove the baking sheet from the oven and let the pork rest for 5 minutes before slicing.

8. Slice the pork tenderloin and serve it alongside the roasted vegetables.

This pork tenderloin and roasted vegetable dish is an excellent diabetes•friendly meal for a college student. The lean pork provides protein, while the variety of vegetables add fiber, vitamins, and minerals. The simple seasoning keeps the dish flavorful without needing to use a lot of salt or sugar.

You can customize the vegetable selection based on your preferences or what's in season. This makes a complete, balanced, and nutritious meal that's easy to prepare.

74. Beef and vegetable kebabs

Ingredient:
- 1 lb beef sirloin or flank steak, cut into 1·inch cubes
- 1 red bell pepper, cut into 1·inch pieces
- 1 zucchini, cut into 1·inch slices
- 1 red onion, cut into 1·inch pieces
- 8 oz mushrooms, halved
- 2 tablespoons olive oil
- 2 tablespoons balsamic vinegar
- 1 teaspoon dried oregano
- 1/2 teaspoon garlic powder
- Salt and pepper to taste
- Wooden or metal skewers

Instructions:
1. In a large bowl, combine the beef cubes, bell pepper, zucchini, onion, and mushrooms.

2. In a small bowl, whisk together the olive oil, balsamic vinegar, oregano, and garlic powder. Pour the marinade over the beef and vegetables and toss to coat.

3. Cover the bowl and refrigerate for 30 minutes to 1 hour, allowing the flavors to meld.

4. Preheat your grill or grill pan to medium·high heat.

5. Thread the marinated beef and vegetables onto the skewers, alternating the ingredients.

6. Grill the kebabs for 12·15 minutes, turning occasionally, until the beef is cooked through and the vegetables are tender.

7. Serve the beef and vegetable kebabs immediately. Enjoy over a bed of cauliflower rice or with a side salad.

These kebabs are a great diabetes·friendly meal option for a college student. The lean beef provides protein, while the vegetables add fiber, vitamins, and minerals. The balsamic marinade adds flavor without needing to use a lot of salt or sugar.

You can customize the vegetables based on your preferences or what's in season. Zucchini, bell peppers, onions, and mushrooms work well, but you could also use cherry tomatoes, eggplant, or asparagus

75. Stuffed bell peppers with ground beef

Ingredient:

- 4 large bell peppers (any color), halved lengthwise and seeds removed
- 1 lb ground beef
- 1 onion, diced
- 3 cloves garlic, minced
- 1 cup cooked cauliflower rice
- 1 (14.5 oz) can diced tomatoes
- 2 tablespoons tomato paste
- 1 teaspoon dried oregano
- 1/2 teaspoon dried basil
- Salt and pepper to taste
- 1/2 cup shredded cheddar cheese (optional)

Instructions:

1. Preheat your oven to 375°F. Lightly grease a baking dish.

2. In a large skillet over medium heat, cook the ground beef until browned and crumbled, 5•7 minutes. Drain any excess fat.

3. Add the diced onion and minced garlic to the skillet. Cook for 3•4 minutes until the onion is translucent.

4. Stir in the cooked cauliflower rice, diced tomatoes, tomato paste, oregano, and basil. Season with salt and pepper to taste.

5. Arrange the bell pepper halves in the prepared baking dish. Spoon the beef and vegetable mixture evenly into the pepper halves.

6. If using, sprinkle the shredded cheddar cheese over the top of the stuffed peppers. Bake for 25•30 minutes, until the peppers are tender and the filling is hot. Serve the stuffed bell peppers immediately.

These stuffed bell peppers are a great diabetes•friendly meal for a college student. The lean ground beef provides protein, while the bell peppers, cauliflower rice, and tomatoes add fiber, vitamins, and minerals. The portion size is appropriate for someone with diabetes.

You can customize the filling by adding other vegetables, herbs, or spices to your liking. Serve the stuffed peppers with a side salad or roasted vegetables for a complete, balanced meal.

76. Pork chops with apple slaw

Ingredient:

Apple Slaw:
• 2 cups shredded green cabbage
• 1 cup shredded red cabbage
• 1 Granny Smith apple, julienned
• 2 tablespoons apple cider vinegar
• 1 tablespoon olive oil
• 1 teaspoon Dijon mustard
• 1 teaspoon honey
• Salt and pepper to taste

Pork Chops:
• 4 (6 oz) boneless pork chops
• 1 tablespoon olive oil
• 1 teaspoon garlic powder
• 1/2 teaspoon dried thyme
• Salt and pepper to taste

Instructions:

1. Preheat your oven to 400°F.

2. Season the pork chops on both sides with the garlic powder, thyme, salt, and pepper.

3. Heat the 1 tablespoon of olive oil in a large oven•safe skillet over medium•high heat.

4. Sear the pork chops for 2•3 minutes per side until browned.

5. Transfer the skillet to the preheated oven and bake the pork chops for 10•12 minutes, until they reach an internal temperature of 145°F.

6. While the pork chops are baking, make the apple slaw. In a large bowl, combine the shredded green and red cabbage, julienned apple, apple cider vinegar, 1 tablespoon olive oil, Dijon mustard, and honey. Toss to coat. Season with salt and pepper. Serve the pork chops immediately, topped with the apple slaw.

This pork chops and apple slaw dish is an excellent diabetes•friendly meal for a college student. The lean pork provides protein, while the apple slaw adds fiber, vitamins, and healthy fats from the olive oil. The portion sizes are appropriate for someone with diabetes.

The flavors of the pork and slaw complement each other nicely, and the recipe is easy to prepare. You can serve this meal with a side of roasted vegetables or a simple salad for a complete, balanced dinner.

77. Beef stew (low-carb version)

Ingredient:

- 1.5 lbs beef stew meat, cut into 1·inch cubes
- 2 tablespoons olive oil
- 1 onion, diced
- 3 cloves garlic, minced
- 2 cups low·sodium beef broth
- 1 (14.5 oz) can diced tomatoes
- 2 bay leaves
- 1 teaspoon dried thyme
- 1/2 teaspoon dried rosemary
- Salt and pepper to taste
- 2 cups cubed zucchini
- 1 cup sliced mushrooms
- 1/4 cup heavy cream (optional)

Instructions:

1. In a large pot or Dutch oven, heat the olive oil over medium·high heat. Add the beef cubes and brown on all sides, about 5 minutes total. Remove the beef from the pot and set aside.

2. Add the diced onion to the pot and sauté for 3·4 minutes until translucent. Add the minced garlic and cook for 1 minute more.

3. Pour in the beef broth and diced tomatoes. Add the bay leaves, thyme, rosemary, and season with salt and pepper.

4. Return the browned beef to the pot and bring the stew to a simmer. Reduce heat to medium·low, cover, and let simmer for 45 minutes.

5. Add the cubed zucchini and sliced mushrooms to the pot. Simmer for an additional 15·20 minutes, until the beef and vegetables are very tender.

6. If desired, stir in the heavy cream during the last 5 minutes of cooking to add a creamy texture.

7. Taste and adjust seasoning as needed. Remove the bay leaves before serving. Serve the low·carb beef stew hot.

This beef stew is a great diabetes·friendly meal for a college student. It's high in protein from the beef, low in carbs by using zucchini instead of potatoes, and full of fiber and nutrients from the vegetables.

78. Pork stir-fry with cabbage

Ingredient:

- 1 lb pork tenderloin, cut into 1•inch pieces
- 2 tablespoons olive oil
- 3 cloves garlic, minced
- 1 tablespoon grated fresh ginger
- 1 head of green cabbage, thinly sliced (about 6 cups)
- 1 red bell pepper, sliced
- 2 tablespoons low•sodium soy sauce
- 1 tablespoon rice vinegar
- 1 teaspoon sesame oil
- Salt and pepper to taste
- Chopped green onions for garnish (optional)

Instructions:

1. In a large skillet or wok, heat the olive oil over high heat.

2. Add the pork pieces and stir•fry for 4•5 minutes until lightly browned on all sides. Remove the pork from the pan and set aside.

3. In the same pan, add the minced garlic and grated ginger. Cook for 1 minute until fragrant.

4. Add the sliced cabbage and bell pepper. Stir•fry for 5•7 minutes, until the vegetables are tender•crisp.

5. Return the cooked pork to the pan. Pour in the soy sauce, rice vinegar, and sesame oil. Toss everything together and cook for 2•3 minutes more, until the pork is cooked through.

6. Season with salt and pepper to taste. Serve the pork and vegetable stir•fry immediately, garnished with chopped green onions if desired.

This pork stir•fry is an excellent diabetes•friendly meal for a college student. The lean pork provides protein, while the cabbage and bell pepper add fiber, vitamins, and minerals. The soy sauce, vinegar, and sesame oil provide lots of flavor without needing to use a lot of salt or sugar.

You can serve this stir•fry over cauliflower rice or zucchini noodles to keep the carbs low. It's a quick, easy, and nutritious meal that's perfect for a busy college student.

79. Beef and mushroom lettuce wraps

Ingredient:

- 1 lb ground beef
- 8 oz sliced mushrooms
- 1 onion, diced
- 3 cloves garlic, minced
- 2 tablespoons low•sodium soy sauce
- 1 tablespoon rice vinegar
- 1 teaspoon sesame oil
- 1/2 teaspoon ground ginger
- 1/4 teaspoon red pepper flakes (optional)
- Salt and pepper to taste
- 1 head of romaine or butter lettuce, leaves separated

Toppings (optional):
- Shredded carrots
- Sliced cucumber
- Chopped green onions
- Chopped cilantro
- Crushed peanuts or cashews

Instructions:

1. In a large skillet or wok, cook the ground beef over medium•high heat, breaking it up with a wooden spoon, until browned and cooked through, about 5•7 minutes. Drain any excess fat.

2. Add the sliced mushrooms, diced onion, and minced garlic to the pan. Cook for 3•4 minutes until the vegetables are tender.

3. Stir in the soy sauce, rice vinegar, sesame oil, ground ginger, and red pepper flakes (if using). Season with salt and pepper to taste.

4. To serve, place a few spoonfuls of the beef and mushroom mixture into the center of a lettuce leaf. Top with any desired toppings. Fold the lettuce leaf over the filling and enjoy.

These beef and mushroom lettuce wraps are a great diabetes•friendly meal. The lean ground beef provides protein, while the mushrooms and lettuce leaves keep the carbs low. The Asian•inspired flavors from the soy sauce, ginger, and sesame oil add lots of taste without needing to use a lot of sugar or salt.

80. BBQ pulled chicken or pork (sugar-free sauce)

Ingredient:

• 2 lbs boneless, skinless chicken breasts or pork shoulder
• 1 cup low•sodium chicken or beef broth
• 1 cup no•sugar•added tomato sauce
• 2 tablespoons apple cider vinegar
• 1 tablespoon Dijon mustard
• 1 teaspoon smoked paprika
• 1 teaspoon garlic powder
• 1/2 teaspoon onion powder
• 1/4 teaspoon cayenne pepper (optional)
• Salt and pepper to taste

Instructions:

1. Place the chicken breasts or pork shoulder in a slow cooker. Pour in the broth.

2. In a small bowl, whisk together the tomato sauce, apple cider vinegar, Dijon mustard, smoked paprika, garlic powder, onion powder, and cayenne pepper (if using). Season with salt and pepper.

3. Pour the sauce mixture over the meat in the slow cooker, making sure the meat is fully coated.

4. Cook on low for 6•8 hours, or on high for 3•4 hours, until the meat is very tender and shreds easily with two forks.

5. Remove the cooked meat from the slow cooker and shred it using two forks.

6. Return the shredded meat to the slow cooker and toss it with the cooking liquid to coat.

7. Serve the sugar•free BBQ pulled chicken or pork on lettuce wraps, over cauliflower rice, or on a bed of steamed vegetables.

This pulled chicken or pork is a great diabetes•friendly meal option for a college student. The meat provides lean protein, while the sugar•free BBQ sauce keeps the carbs and sugar low.

You can customize the spices and seasonings to your taste. Serve the pulled meat with a side salad, roasted veggies, or a small portion of whole grain rolls or buns for a complete meal.

81. Steamed broccoli with lemon

Ingredient:

- 1 lb broccoli florets
- 2 tablespoons water
- 1 tablespoon fresh lemon juice
- 1 teaspoon olive oil
- Salt and pepper to taste

Instructions:

1. Place the broccoli florets in a steamer basket set over a pot of simmering water. Cover and steam for 5•7 minutes, until the broccoli is tender•crisp.

2. Transfer the steamed broccoli to a serving bowl.

3. Drizzle the lemon juice and olive oil over the broccoli. Toss gently to coat.

4. Season the broccoli with salt and pepper to taste.

5. Serve the steamed broccoli with lemon immediately.

This is a simple, diabetes•friendly side dish that's perfect for a college student. Broccoli is high in fiber, vitamins, and minerals, making it a nutritious vegetable choice.

The lemon juice and olive oil add bright, fresh flavor without needing to use any high•sodium or sugary sauces or seasonings. This preparation allows the natural taste of the broccoli to shine.

You can customize this recipe by adding a sprinkle of grated Parmesan cheese, a pinch of garlic powder, or some chopped fresh herbs like parsley or basil.

Steamed broccoli with lemon makes a great accompaniment to grilled or baked chicken, fish, or pork. It's an easy, healthy side that's quick to prepare.

82. Roasted Brussels sprouts with bacon

Ingredient:

- 1 lb Brussels sprouts, trimmed and halved
- 2 tablespoons olive oil
- 1/4 teaspoon salt
- 1/4 teaspoon black pepper
- 4 slices bacon, cooked until crispy and crumbled

Instructions:

1. Preheat your oven to 400°F. Line a baking sheet with parchment paper.

2. In a large bowl, toss the Brussels sprouts with the olive oil, salt, and pepper until evenly coated.

3. Spread the Brussels sprouts in a single layer on the prepared baking sheet.

4. Roast for 20•25 minutes, tossing halfway, until the Brussels sprouts are tender and lightly browned.

5. Remove the roasted Brussels sprouts from the oven and transfer to a serving bowl.

6. Sprinkle the crumbled bacon over the top.

7. Serve the roasted Brussels sprouts with bacon immediately.

This roasted Brussels sprouts dish is an excellent diabetes•friendly side. Brussels sprouts are high in fiber, vitamins, and minerals, while the bacon adds a delicious savory flavor.

The portion size is appropriate for someone with diabetes, and the recipe doesn't require any added sugars or high•sodium ingredients. It's a simple, nutritious, and tasty way for a college student to enjoy their veggies.

You can customize this recipe by adding other spices or herbs, such as garlic powder, paprika, or parmesan cheese. Serve it alongside grilled chicken, fish, or a lean protein for a complete, balanced meal.

83. Cauliflower mash

Ingredient:

- 1 large head of cauliflower, cut into florets (about 4 cups)
- 2 tbsp unsalted butter
- 2 tbsp milk or unsweetened almond milk
- 1/4 cup grated Parmesan cheese (optional)
- Salt and pepper to taste

Instructions:

1. In a large pot, bring 1·2 inches of water to a boil. Add the cauliflower florets, cover, and steam for 10·12 minutes, until very tender.

2. Drain the steamed cauliflower well and transfer it to a food processor or high·powered blender.

3. Add the butter, milk, and Parmesan cheese (if using) to the food processor. Blend or process until the mixture is smooth and creamy, scraping down the sides as needed.

4. Season the cauliflower mash with salt and pepper to taste.

5. Serve the cauliflower mash warm, garnished with additional Parmesan cheese, chopped chives, or a drizzle of olive oil if desired.

Tips:
- For a creamier texture, add an extra tablespoon or two of milk.

- Roast the cauliflower florets before mashing for a deeper, more caramelized flavor.

- Experiment with different herbs and spices, such as garlic powder, onion powder, or fresh thyme.

- This cauliflower mash can be a great low·carb alternative to traditional mashed potatoes.

- Reheat leftovers gently on the stovetop or in the microwave, adding a splash of milk if needed to maintain the desired consistency.

Enjoy this simple, versatile, and nutritious cauliflower mash!

84. Quinoa pilaf with herbs

Ingredient:
- 1 cup uncooked quinoa, rinsed
- 2 cups low•sodium vegetable or chicken broth
- 1 tbsp olive oil
- 1 small onion, diced
- 2 cloves garlic, minced
- 1/4 cup chopped fresh parsley
- 2 tbsp chopped fresh basil
- 1 tbsp chopped fresh thyme
- Salt and pepper to taste

Instructions:

1. In a medium saucepan, combine the rinsed quinoa and broth. Bring to a boil over high heat.

2. Once boiling, reduce the heat to low, cover the saucepan, and simmer for 15•20 minutes, until the quinoa is tender and the liquid is absorbed.

3. Remove the saucepan from the heat and let the quinoa sit, covered, for 5 minutes.

4. In a large skillet, heat the olive oil over medium heat. Add the diced onion and sauté for 3•4 minutes, until translucent.

5. Add the minced garlic to the skillet and cook for 1 minute, until fragrant.

6. Fluff the cooked quinoa with a fork and add it to the skillet with the onions and garlic. Stir to combine.

7. Remove the skillet from the heat and stir in the chopped parsley, basil, and thyme. Season with salt and pepper to taste.

8. Serve the quinoa pilaf warm, garnished with additional fresh herbs if desired.

Tips:
- Use a variety of fresh herbs for maximum flavor.
- Toasted nuts or dried cranberries can also be added for extra texture and flavor.
- Quinoa is a great source of protein, fiber, and complex carbohydrates.
- This pilaf can be served as a main dish or a side.

85. Sauteed spinach with garlic

Ingredient:

• 1 lb fresh spinach, washed and stems removed
• 1 tbsp olive oil
• 3 cloves garlic, minced
• 1/4 tsp red pepper flakes (optional)
• Salt and pepper to taste

Instructions:

1. In a large skillet or wok, heat the olive oil over medium heat.

2. Add the minced garlic and sauté for 1•2 minutes, until fragrant, being careful not to let the garlic burn.

3. Add the fresh spinach to the skillet in batches, if needed, and sauté for 2•3 minutes, stirring frequently, until the spinach is wilted and tender.

4. If using, sprinkle the red pepper flakes over the sautéed spinach.

5. Season with salt and pepper to taste.

6. Serve the sautéed spinach with garlic warm.

Tips for a college student with diabetes:
• Spinach is an excellent source of vitamins, minerals, and fiber, making it a great choice for a diabetic•friendly side dish.
• The small amount of olive oil provides healthy fats without significantly increasing the carbohydrate content.
• Garlic is a flavorful addition that doesn't add any carbs.
• The red pepper flakes are optional, but they can add a nice kick of flavor and potential health benefits.
• Pair this sautéed spinach with a lean protein, such as grilled chicken or baked fish, for a balanced meal.
• Drink water or unsweetened tea instead of sugary beverages.
• Monitor your blood sugar levels and adjust your insulin dosage accordingly.

This simple, nutrient•dense sautéed spinach dish is a great option for a college student with diabetes, providing essential vitamins and minerals without a significant impact on blood sugar levels.

86. Green beans almondine

Ingredient:

- 1 lb fresh green beans, trimmed
- 2 tbsp unsalted butter
- 1/4 cup sliced almonds
- 1 tbsp lemon juice
- Salt and pepper to taste

Instructions:

1. Bring a large pot of salted water to a boil. Add the green beans and cook for 3•5 minutes, until tender•crisp. Drain and rinse with cold water to stop the cooking.

2. In a skillet, melt the butter over medium heat. Add the sliced almonds and cook, stirring frequently, until the almonds are lightly toasted, about 2•3 minutes.

3. Add the cooked green beans to the skillet with the toasted almonds. Toss to coat the beans in the butter and almonds.

4. Drizzle the lemon juice over the green beans and almonds. Season with salt and pepper to taste.

5. Serve the green beans almondine warm. Enjoy!

The key is to lightly cook the green beans until tender•crisp, then toss them with the toasted almonds and lemon butter sauce. This simple side dish is a classic French•inspired preparation that brings out the fresh flavor of the green beans.

87. Roasted sweet potatoes (in moderation)

Ingredient:

- 2 medium sweet potatoes, peeled and cut into 1•inch cubes (about 2 cups cubed)
- 1 tbsp olive oil
- 1 tsp ground cinnamon
- 1/4 tsp ground nutmeg
- Salt and pepper to taste

Instructions:

1. Preheat your oven to 400°F (200°C).

2. In a large bowl, toss the cubed sweet potatoes with the olive oil, cinnamon, nutmeg, salt, and pepper until the potatoes are evenly coated.

3. Spread the seasoned sweet potato cubes in a single layer on a baking sheet lined with parchment paper.

4. Roast the sweet potatoes for 20•25 minutes, flipping halfway through, until they are tender and lightly browned.

5. Remove the roasted sweet potatoes from the oven and serve warm.

Tips:
- For a small portion, use 2 medium sweet potatoes, which will yield about 2 cups of roasted cubes.
- Adjust the cooking time as needed, depending on the size of your potato cubes.
- You can also add other spices like garlic powder, paprika, or chili powder to the seasoning mix.
- Toss the roasted sweet potatoes with a bit of maple syrup or honey for a touch of sweetness.
- Serve the roasted sweet potatoes as a side dish or add them to salads, grain bowls, or other meals.

Enjoy these flavorful, nutrient•dense roasted sweet potatoes in moderation as part of a balanced diet.

88. Cucumber and tomato salad

Ingredient:

- 2 medium cucumbers, sliced
- 2 cups cherry or grape tomatoes, halved
- 1/2 red onion, thinly sliced
- 2 tbsp fresh chopped parsley
- 2 tbsp olive oil
- 1 tbsp red wine vinegar
- 1 tsp Dijon mustard
- Salt and pepper to taste

Instructions:

1. In a large bowl, combine the sliced cucumbers, halved tomatoes, and thinly sliced red onion.

2. In a small bowl, whisk together the olive oil, red wine vinegar, Dijon mustard, salt, and pepper.

3. Pour the dressing over the cucumber and tomato mixture and toss gently to coat.

4. Sprinkle the fresh chopped parsley over the top.

5. Cover and refrigerate for at least 30 minutes to allow the flavors to meld.

6. Serve chilled or at room temperature.

Tips:
- For best flavor, use fresh, ripe tomatoes and crisp cucumbers.
- You can substitute balsamic vinegar for the red wine vinegar if desired.
- Add a pinch of sugar to the dressing if your tomatoes are a bit tart.
- Garnish with crumbled feta cheese or sliced black olives.

This simple cucumber and tomato salad makes a refreshing side dish or light lunch. The tangy vinaigrette complements the fresh veggies perfectly.

89. Steamed asparagus with Parmesan

Ingredient:

- 1 lb fresh asparagus, trimmed
- 1 tbsp unsalted butter
- 2 tbsp grated Parmesan cheese
- Salt and pepper to taste

Instructions:

1. Fill a medium saucepan with about 1 inch of water and bring it to a boil over high heat.

2. Add the trimmed asparagus spears to the saucepan. Cover and steam for 5•7 minutes, until the asparagus is tender•crisp.

3. Carefully remove the steamed asparagus from the saucepan and transfer it to a serving dish.

4. In a small microwave•safe bowl, melt the butter. Drizzle the melted butter over the steamed asparagus.

5. Sprinkle the grated Parmesan cheese evenly over the asparagus.

6. Season with salt and pepper to taste.

7. Serve the steamed asparagus with Parmesan immediately, while hot.

Tips for a college student with diabetes:
- Steaming the asparagus is a healthy cooking method that preserves nutrients without adding extra fat or calories.
- The small portion of Parmesan cheese provides flavor without significantly increasing the carbohydrate or calorie content.
- Pair this dish with a lean protein, such as grilled chicken or baked fish, for a balanced meal.
- Drink water or unsweetened tea instead of sugary beverages.
- Monitor your blood sugar levels and adjust your insulin dosage accordingly.

This simple, nutrient•dense side dish is a great option for a college student with diabetes, providing fiber, vitamins, and a touch of indulgence from the Parmesan cheese.

90. Grilled corn on the cob (small portion)

Ingredient:
• 2 ears of fresh corn, husks and silk removed
• 2 tbsp unsalted butter, softened
• Salt and pepper to taste

Instructions:

1. Preheat your grill to medium·high heat.

2. Spread the softened butter evenly over the corn cobs. Season with salt and pepper.

3. Place the corn directly on the grill grates. Grill for 10·12 minutes, rotating the cobs occasionally, until the kernels are tender and lightly charred.

4. Remove the corn from the grill and let it cool for a minute or two.

5. Serve the grilled corn on the cob warm, with any additional butter, salt, and pepper on the side if desired.

Tips:
• For a small portion, 2 ears of corn should be enough for 1·2 people.

• Soak the corn in water for 30 minutes before grilling to help steam the kernels.

• You can also brush the corn with a bit of olive oil or melted butter before seasoning.

• Experiment with different seasonings like chili powder, garlic powder, or Parmesan cheese.

Enjoy this simple, delicious grilled corn on the cob! The high heat of the grill brings out the natural sweetness of the corn.

91. Sugar-free Jello with whipped cream

Ingredient:

- 1 (3 oz) package sugar•free Jello (any flavor)
- 2 cups water
- 1 cup unsweetened almond milk or low•fat milk
- 1 cup heavy whipping cream
- 1 tsp vanilla extract
- 1•2 tbsp granulated erythritol or other zero•calorie sweetener (optional)

Instructions:

1. In a medium saucepan, bring the 2 cups of water to a boil. Remove from heat and stir in the sugar•free Jello powder until dissolved.

2. Pour the Jello mixture into a 4•6 cup mold or individual ramekins. Refrigerate for at least 4 hours, or until set.

3. In a medium bowl, use a hand mixer or stand mixer to whip the heavy cream until it forms soft peaks. Add the vanilla extract and 1•2 tablespoons of granulated erythritol or other zero•calorie sweetener, if desired, and continue whipping until the cream is stiff.

4. Unmold the set Jello and top with the sweetened whipped cream.

5. Serve chilled.

Tips for a College Student with Diabetes:

• Choose a sugar•free Jello flavor that you enjoy, such as strawberry, raspberry, or lemon.

• The unsweetened almond milk or low•fat milk helps create a creamy texture without adding too many carbs.

• The heavy whipping cream provides a rich, indulgent topping, but you can use a lower•fat whipped topping if preferred.

• The optional erythritol or other zero•calorie sweetener can add a touch of sweetness to the whipped cream without affecting blood sugar levels.

• Portion control is key • a small serving of this dessert can be a satisfying treat.

• Pair this with a protein•rich snack, such as a hard•boiled egg or a small serving of nuts, for a more balanced option.

92. Berries with Greek yogurt

Ingredient:

• 1 cup fresh or frozen mixed berries (such as blueberries, raspberries, and blackberries)
• 1 cup plain, unsweetened Greek yogurt
• 1 tsp honey (optional)

Instructions:

1. In a medium bowl, gently mix the fresh or frozen berries with the plain, unsweetened Greek yogurt.

2. If desired, drizzle the mixture with 1 tsp of honey for a touch of sweetness.

3. Serve the berries and Greek yogurt immediately, or refrigerate until ready to serve.

Tips for a College Student with Diabetes:

• Berries are an excellent source of fiber, vitamins, and antioxidants, and they have a relatively low glycemic index, making them a diabetes•friendly fruit choice.

• Greek yogurt is high in protein and low in carbohydrates, which can help slow the absorption of the natural sugars in the berries.

• The optional honey provides a small amount of sweetness, but you can omit it if you prefer a less sweet dish.

• Avoid flavored or sweetened yogurts, as they often contain added sugars that can spike blood sugar levels.

• Pair this dish with a lean protein, such as a hard•boiled egg or a small serving of nuts, for a balanced snack or light meal.

• Drink water or unsweetened tea instead of sugary beverages.

• Monitor your blood sugar levels and adjust your insulin dosage accordingly.

This simple, nutrient•dense combination of berries and Greek yogurt is an excellent choice for a college student with diabetes, providing a satisfying and diabetes•friendly treat or snack.

93. Dark chocolate (70% cocoa or higher)

Ingredient:

- 2 cups heavy whipping cream
- 1 cup unsweetened almond milk (or regular milk)
- 1/2 cup granulated erythritol or other zero•calorie sweetener
- 1 tsp vanilla extract
- 1/8 tsp salt

Instructions:

1. In a medium bowl, combine the heavy whipping cream, almond milk (or regular milk), erythritol, vanilla extract, and salt. Whisk until the sweetener is fully dissolved.

2. Pour the mixture into an ice cream maker and churn according to the manufacturer's instructions, usually 20•30 minutes.

3. Once the ice cream has reached your desired consistency, transfer it to an airtight container and place it in the freezer for at least 2 hours before serving.

4. Scoop and serve the sugar•free ice cream as desired.

Tips:
- For a creamier texture, use a higher ratio of heavy cream to milk.

- Experiment with different zero•calorie sweeteners like xylitol or monk fruit sweetener.

- Add mix•ins like chopped nuts, sugar•free chocolate chips, or fresh berries.

- Allow the ice cream to sit at room temperature for 5•10 minutes before scooping for a softer texture.

- Store the ice cream in an airtight container in the freezer for up to 2 months.

This sugar•free ice cream is a great option for a college student with diabetes, as it satisfies the craving for a sweet treat without the added sugar. Be sure to monitor your portion sizes and blood sugar levels when enjoying this homemade dessert.

94. Sugar-free ice cream or gelato

Ingredient:

- 2 cups unsweetened almond milk
- 1 cup heavy cream
- 1/2 cup granulated erythritol or other zero•calorie sweetener
- 1 tsp vanilla extract
- 1/8 tsp salt

Instructions:

1. In a medium saucepan, combine the almond milk, heavy cream, erythritol, vanilla extract, and salt. Whisk the ingredients together and heat over medium, stirring frequently, until the sweetener has dissolved and the mixture is hot but not boiling, about 5 minutes.

2. Remove the saucepan from the heat and let the mixture cool to room temperature, about 30 minutes.

3. Once cooled, transfer the mixture to a blender and blend until smooth and creamy.

4. Pour the gelato base into an ice cream maker and churn according to the manufacturer's instructions, usually 20•30 minutes.

5. Once the gelato has reached your desired consistency, transfer it to an airtight container and place it in the freezer for at least 2 hours before serving. Scoop and serve the sugar•free gelato as desired.

Tips:
- For a richer, creamier gelato, use a higher ratio of heavy cream to almond milk.

- Experiment with different zero•calorie sweeteners like xylitol or monk fruit sweetener.

- Add mix•ins like chopped nuts, sugar•free chocolate chips, or fresh berries.

- Allow the gelato to sit at room temperature for 5•10 minutes before scooping for a softer texture. Store the gelato in an airtight container in the freezer for up to 2 months.

This sugar•free gelato is a great option for a college student with diabetes, as it provides a creamy, indulgent treat without the added sugar. Be sure to monitor your portion sizes and blood sugar levels when enjoying this homemade dessert.

95. Coconut macaroons

Ingredient:

- 2 cups unsweetened shredded coconut
- 1/4 cup granulated erythritol or other zero•calorie sweetener
- 2 large egg whites
- 1/4 tsp vanilla extract
- 1/8 tsp salt

Instructions:

1. Preheat your oven to 325°F (165°C). Line a baking sheet with parchment paper.

2. In a medium bowl, combine the unsweetened shredded coconut and granulated erythritol (or other zero•calorie sweetener). Mix well to distribute the sweetener evenly.

3. In a separate small bowl, beat the egg whites until they are foamy and form soft peaks.

4. Add the vanilla extract and salt to the beaten egg whites, and continue beating until the egg whites are stiff and glossy.

5. Gently fold the whipped egg whites into the coconut mixture until well combined.

6. Scoop the coconut macaroon mixture by the tablespoonful onto the prepared baking sheet, spacing them about 1 inch apart.

7. Bake the macaroons for 15•18 minutes, or until the edges are lightly golden brown.

8. Remove the baking sheet from the oven and let the macaroons cool on the sheet for 5 minutes before transferring them to a wire rack to cool completely.

Tips:
• Use a zero•calorie sweetener like erythritol, xylitol, or monk fruit sweetener to keep these macaroons sugar•free.
• For a chewier texture, bake the macaroons for the shorter end of the time range.
• For a crunchier exterior, bake them for the longer end of the time range.
• Store the cooled macaroons in an airtight container at room temperature for up to 1 week.

Enjoy these delicious, sugar•free coconut macaroons as a guilt•free treat!

96. Baked apples with cinnamon

Ingredient:

- 4 medium·sized apples (such as Gala, Honeycrisp, or Fuji)
- 1/4 cup (60ml) unsweetened apple juice or water
- 2 tbsp (30ml) granulated erythritol or monk fruit sweetener
- 1 tsp ground cinnamon
- 1/4 tsp ground nutmeg (optional)
- 2 tbsp (30g) chopped walnuts or pecans (optional)

Instructions:

1. Preheat the oven to 375°F (190°C).

2. Core the apples, leaving the bottom intact so they can stand upright. Use a paring knife or melon baller to scoop out the core, creating a well in the center of each apple.

3. Place the cored apples in a baking dish and pour the apple juice or water into the bottom of the dish.

4. In a small bowl, mix together the erythritol, cinnamon, and nutmeg (if using). Spoon this mixture into the center of each apple.

5. If using, sprinkle the chopped nuts over the top of the apples.

6. Bake for 30·40 minutes, or until the apples are tender when pierced with a fork. Baste the apples with the juices in the baking dish a few times during baking.

7. Serve the baked apples warm, with the juices from the baking dish spooned over the top.

These baked apples are a great source of fiber, vitamins, and antioxidants. The cinnamon and erythritol provide sweetness without spiking blood sugar levels. This makes a delicious and healthy dessert or snack for a college student with diabetes.

97. Peanut butter cookies

Ingredient:

- 1 cup (256g) creamy peanut butter (make sure it's just peanuts and salt)
- 3/4 cup (90g) granulated erythritol or monk fruit sweetener
- 1 large egg
- 1 tsp vanilla extract
- 1/4 tsp salt

Instructions:

1. Preheat the oven to 350°F (177°C). Line a baking sheet with parchment paper.

2. In a medium bowl, stir together the peanut butter, erythritol, egg, vanilla, and salt until well combined.

3. Scoop rounded tablespoons of the dough and place them about 2 inches apart on the prepared baking sheet. Use a fork to gently press a criss•cross pattern on the top of each cookie.

4. Bake for 8•10 minutes, until the edges are lightly golden. Be careful not to overbake.

5. Allow the cookies to cool on the baking sheet for 5 minutes before transferring them to a wire rack to cool completely.

These sugar•free peanut butter cookies are soft, chewy, and satisfying. The erythritol provides sweetness without affecting blood sugar levels. Peanut butter is a great source of protein, healthy fats, and fiber, making these cookies a nutritious treat for a college student with diabetes.

Store the cookies in an airtight container at room temperature for up to 1 week. Enjoy!

98. Almond flour brownies

Ingredient:

- 1 cup (112g) almond flour
- 1/4 cup (20g) unsweetened cocoa powder
- 1/4 tsp salt
- 1/4 tsp baking soda
- 1/2 cup (120ml) unsweetened almond milk
- 1/3 cup (80ml) melted coconut oil or unsalted butter
- 1/2 cup (120ml) granulated erythritol or monk fruit sweetener
- 1 tsp vanilla extract
- 2 large eggs

Instructions:

1. Preheat the oven to 350°F (177°C). Grease an 8x8 inch baking pan.

2. In a medium bowl, whisk together the almond flour, cocoa powder, salt, and baking soda.

3. In a separate bowl, whisk together the almond milk, melted coconut oil, erythritol, and vanilla. Then whisk in the eggs until fully incorporated.

4. Pour the wet ingredients into the dry ingredients and stir just until combined, being careful not to overmix.

5. Spread the batter evenly into the prepared baking pan.

6. Bake for 18•22 minutes, until a toothpick inserted in the center comes out clean.

7. Allow the brownies to cool completely in the pan before cutting into squares.

These sugar•free almond flour brownies are rich, fudgy, and low in carbs. The almond flour provides healthy fats and fiber, while the erythritol sweetens them without spiking blood sugar. They make a great treat for a college student with diabetes.

99. Chia seed pudding with cocoa

Ingredient:

- 1/4 cup (40g) chia seeds
- 1 cup (240ml) unsweetened almond milk
- 2 tbsp (10g) unsweetened cocoa powder
- 1•2 tbsp (15•30ml) granulated erythritol or monk fruit sweetener (to taste)
- 1 tsp vanilla extract
- Pinch of salt

Instructions:

1. In a medium bowl, whisk together the chia seeds, almond milk, cocoa powder, erythritol, vanilla, and salt until well combined.

2. Cover the bowl and refrigerate for at least 2 hours, or overnight, stirring occasionally, until the mixture has thickened to a pudding•like consistency.

3. Taste and adjust sweetener if desired. The chia seeds will continue to thicken the pudding as it sits.

4. Serve chilled, topped with fresh berries, chopped nuts, or a dollop of unsweetened whipped cream if desired.

This chia seed pudding is high in fiber, protein, and healthy fats from the chia seeds and almond milk. The cocoa powder provides a rich chocolate flavor without added sugar. The erythritol sweetens it without spiking blood sugar levels.

This makes a great breakfast, snack, or dessert option for a college student with diabetes. It's easy to prepare ahead of time and can be customized with different toppings.

100. Avocado chocolate mousse

Ingredient:

- 2 ripe avocados, pitted and flesh scooped out
- 1/4 cup unsweetened cocoa powder
- 1/4 cup unsweetened almond milk (or milk of choice)
- 2•3 tbsp granulated erythritol or stevia (to taste)
- 1 tsp vanilla extract
- Pinch of salt

Instructions:

1. In a food processor or high•powered blender, combine the avocado flesh, cocoa powder, almond milk, erythritol/stevia, vanilla, and salt. Blend until smooth and creamy.

2. Taste and adjust sweetener as needed. The avocado provides creaminess while the cocoa powder gives it a rich chocolate flavor.

3. Spoon the mousse into individual serving dishes or ramekins. Refrigerate for at least 30 minutes before serving to allow it to set.

4. Top with a sprinkle of cocoa powder, chopped nuts, or fresh berries if desired.

This recipe is low in carbs and sugar, high in healthy fats from the avocado, and provides a satisfying chocolate treat. The avocado also adds fiber, vitamins, and minerals. It's a great option for a college student with diabetes looking for a healthier dessert.

101. Water with lemon or cucumber slices

Ingredient:

- 1 liter (4 cups) of cold water
- 1 lemon, sliced

OR

- 1 cucumber, sliced

Instructions:

1. Fill a pitcher or water bottle with the cold water.

2. Add the lemon or cucumber slices to the water.

3. Refrigerate for at least 2 hours, or up to 24 hours, to allow the flavors to infuse the water.

4. Serve the infused water chilled, with the lemon or cucumber slices still in the pitcher.

Tips:
- You can use a combination of lemon and cucumber slices for a more complex flavor.

- Try adding a few sprigs of fresh herbs like mint, basil, or rosemary for extra flavor.

- Refill the pitcher with more water as you drink it to continue extracting the flavors.

- The longer you let it infuse, the stronger the flavor will be.

- Infused waters are a great way to stay hydrated and add natural flavor without added sugars.

102. Herbal teas (unsweetened)

Ingredient:
- 1•2 tablespoons fresh lemon balm leaves
- 1 cup boiling water
- Honey or lemon (optional)

Instructions:

1. Rinse the fresh lemon balm leaves and gently pat dry.

2. Place the lemon balm leaves in a teapot or heatproof mug.

3. Pour the boiling water over the leaves and let steep for 5•7 minutes.

4. Strain the tea leaves out using a fine mesh strainer or tea infuser.

5. Optionally, stir in a teaspoon or two of honey or a squeeze of fresh lemon juice to taste.

6. Enjoy the soothing, lemony flavor of the lemon balm tea.

Tips:
- Use 1•2 tablespoons of fresh lemon balm per cup of water, depending on how strong you want the flavor.

- Lemon balm has a calming effect, so this tea can be enjoyed any time of day.

- You can also dry the lemon balm leaves and store them to make tea later.

103. Sparkling water with a splash of lime

Ingredient:

• 1 cup (8 oz) chilled sparkling water
• 1•2 tablespoons freshly squeezed lime juice

Instructions:

1. Fill a glass with chilled sparkling water.

2. Add 1•2 tablespoons of freshly squeezed lime juice, to taste. Start with 1 tablespoon and add more if desired.

3. Stir gently to combine.

4. Serve immediately over ice, if desired.

Tips:

• Use freshly squeezed lime juice for the best flavor. Avoid using bottled lime juice.

• You can also add a lime wedge or slice as a garnish.

• For a little extra flavor, you can add a few mint leaves or a small slice of lime peel.

• This is a refreshing and hydrating beverage that's perfect for hot days or anytime you want a flavorful sparkling drink without added sugars.

• Feel free to experiment with other citrus juices like lemon, orange, or grapefruit as well.

104. Unsweetened almond milk or soy milk

Ingredient:
• 1 cup raw almonds or soybeans
• 4 cups filtered water
• Pinch of salt (optional)

Instructions for Almond Milk:

1. Soak the raw almonds in water for 8•12 hours or overnight. This helps soften them.

2. Drain and rinse the soaked almonds.

3. Add the almonds and 4 cups of fresh filtered water to a high•powered blender. Blend on high for 1•2 minutes until very smooth.

4. Strain the almond milk through a nut milk bag or fine mesh strainer to remove the pulp.

5. Stir in a pinch of salt if desired.

6. Store the unsweetened almond milk in an airtight container in the refrigerator for up to 4•5 days.

Instructions for Soy Milk:

1. Soak the soybeans in water for 8•12 hours or overnight. Drain and rinse.

2. Add the soaked soybeans and 4 cups of fresh filtered water to a blender. Blend on high for 2•3 minutes until very smooth.

3. Pour the soy milk mixture into a pot and heat over medium, stirring frequently, until it just starts to simmer.

4. Remove from heat and strain through a fine mesh strainer to remove the okara (soy pulp).

5. Stir in a pinch of salt if desired.

6. Store the unsweetened soy milk in an airtight container in the refrigerator for up to 4•5 days.

Enjoy your homemade unsweetened plant•based milk!

105. Coffee or tea (black or with sugar-free sweetener)

Ingredient:
• 1 cup brewed coffee
• 1•2 packets of sugar•free sweetener (such as stevia, monk fruit, or erythritol)
• Optional: Unsweetened almond milk or soy milk

Instructions:
1. Brew a cup of coffee.

2. Add 1•2 packets of your preferred sugar•free sweetener and stir to dissolve.

3. If desired, add a splash of unsweetened almond milk or soy milk.

Tea with Sugar•Free Sweetener

Ingredients:
• 1 cup brewed black, green, or herbal tea
• 1•2 packets of sugar•free sweetener
• Optional: Lemon wedge

Instructions:
1. Brew a cup of your favorite tea.

2. Add 1•2 packets of sugar•free sweetener and stir to dissolve.

3. Optionally, add a squeeze of fresh lemon juice.

Tips:
• Start with 1 packet of sweetener and add more to taste. Some sugar•free sweeteners can have a stronger flavor.

• Unsweetened almond milk or soy milk can add creaminess to coffee or tea.

• Experiment with different sugar•free sweeteners to find your preferred taste.

• Herbal teas like chamomile or peppermint can also be enjoyed with sugar•free sweeteners.

106. Vegetable juices (low-sodium)

Ingredient:

- 2 carrots, peeled
- 1 cucumber
- 2 celery stalks
- 1 cup spinach or kale
- 1/2 green apple (optional)
- 1·inch piece of ginger (optional)
- Filtered water (if needed)

Instructions:

1. Wash all the vegetables thoroughly.

2. Cut the carrots, cucumber, celery, and apple (if using) into pieces that will fit through your juicer chute.

3. Add the vegetables and ginger (if using) to your juicer and juice according to the manufacturer's instructions.

4. If the juice is very thick, you can thin it out with a small amount of filtered water.

5. Pour the juice into a glass and enjoy immediately.

Tips:

- Use organic produce when possible to avoid pesticide residues.

- Adjust the ingredient amounts to your taste preferences. You can use more greens for a more vegetal flavor.

- Avoid adding salt to keep the sodium content low.

- Store any leftover juice in an airtight container in the refrigerator for up to 3 days.

- You can also freeze the juice in ice cube trays for easy portioning later.

- This juice is packed with vitamins, minerals, and antioxidants from the vegetables.

107. Green tea with ginger

Ingredient:

- 1 cup (8 oz) freshly boiled water
- 1•2 teaspoons loose leaf green tea or 1 green tea bag
- 1•inch piece of fresh ginger, peeled and sliced

Instructions:

1. Bring the water to a boil in a small saucepan or kettle.

2. Place the green tea leaves or tea bag in a teapot or heatproof mug.

3. Slice the fresh ginger and add it to the teapot or mug.

4. Pour the boiling water over the tea and ginger.

5. Allow the tea to steep for 3•5 minutes.

6. Remove the tea leaves or bag and ginger slices.

7. Pour the brewed green tea into a cup and enjoy.

Tips:

- Use high•quality, fresh green tea for the best flavor.

- Adjust the amount of ginger to your taste preference. Start with 1•inch and add more if you want a stronger ginger flavor.

- You can also grate the ginger instead of slicing it if you prefer a more intense ginger taste.

- For an extra boost of flavor, you can add a squeeze of fresh lemon juice or a drizzle of honey.

- Drink the green tea with ginger hot or chilled over ice.

The combination of the earthy green tea and the spicy, aromatic ginger makes for a soothing and refreshing beverage. Enjoy!

108. Protein shakes (low–sugar)

Ingredient:

• 1 scoop (about 25•30g) unflavored or vanilla protein powder
• 1 cup unsweetened almond milk or unsweetened soy milk
• 1/2 cup frozen berries (such as blueberries, raspberries, or strawberries)
• 1 tablespoon nut butter (such as almond or peanut butter)
• 1/2 teaspoon vanilla extract (optional)
• 1•2 ice cubes (optional)

Instructions:

1. Add all the ingredients to a high•powered blender.

2. Blend on high speed until smooth and creamy, about 30•60 seconds.

3. Pour the protein shake into a glass and enjoy immediately.

Tips for a Low•Sugar Protein Shake:

• Choose an unflavored or vanilla protein powder, as flavored powders often contain added sugars.

• Use unsweetened plant•based milks like almond or soy milk instead of dairy milk, which has natural sugars.

• Stick to 1/2 cup of frozen berries, which provide natural sweetness without too much sugar.

• Avoid adding honey, maple syrup, or other sweeteners.

• You can also use fresh spinach or kale for extra nutrients without adding sugar.

Nutritional Information (per serving):
• Calories: 250•300
• Protein: 20•25g
• Carbs: 15•20g
• Sugar: 5•10g

This low•sugar protein shake is a great way to get a nutritious, filling snack or meal replacement. Adjust the ingredients to your taste preferences.

109. Kombucha (low-sugar varieties)

Ingredient:

• 4 cups brewed black or green tea, cooled to room temperature
• 1/2 cup organic cane sugar or honey
• 1 kombucha SCOBY (Symbiotic Culture of Bacteria and Yeast)
• 1 cup unflavored kombucha from a previous batch (or store•bought)

Instructions:

1. In a large glass or ceramic container, combine the cooled tea and sugar/honey. Stir until the sugar/honey is fully dissolved.

2. Gently add the SCOBY and the 1 cup of unflavored kombucha. Cover the container with a coffee filter or breathable cloth and secure it with a rubber band.

3. Allow the kombucha to ferment at room temperature (70•85°F) for 7•14 days, checking it periodically. The longer it ferments, the less sweet it will become as the yeast and bacteria convert the sugar.

4. Once it reaches your desired level of sweetness and fizziness, remove the SCOBY and 1 cup of the kombucha to use as a starter for your next batch.

5. Transfer the remaining kombucha to bottles or jars and refrigerate. It will continue to develop more carbonation as it chills.

Tips for Low•Sugar Kombucha:

• Use less sugar (1/4 to 1/2 cup per 4 cups of tea) for a lower sugar content.
• Ferment for 10•14 days to allow more of the sugar to be consumed.
• Avoid adding fruit juices or other sweeteners, which will increase the sugar content.
• Look for low•sugar commercial kombucha varieties (under 6g sugar per serving).

110. Tomato juice (low-sodium)

Ingredient:
• 4 lbs ripe tomatoes, cored and quartered
• 1 cup water
• 1 tablespoon lemon juice
• 1/4 teaspoon black pepper
• 1/8 teaspoon cayenne pepper (optional)

Instructions:

1. In a large pot, combine the quartered tomatoes and 1 cup of water. Bring to a boil over medium•high heat.

2. Reduce the heat to medium•low and simmer the tomatoes for 20•25 minutes, stirring occasionally, until they are very soft.

3. Remove the pot from the heat and let the tomato mixture cool slightly.

4. Working in batches, carefully transfer the tomato mixture to a blender or food processor. Blend until smooth.

5. Strain the blended tomato mixture through a fine mesh sieve or cheesecloth to remove any seeds and skins. Discard the solids.

6. Stir in the lemon juice, black pepper, and cayenne pepper (if using).

7. Taste and adjust seasoning as needed. Add more lemon juice for acidity or pepper for spice.

8. Pour the low•sodium tomato juice into a pitcher or jars and refrigerate until ready to serve.

Tips:
• Use ripe, in•season tomatoes for the best flavor.
• Avoid adding salt to keep the sodium content low.
• Serve the tomato juice chilled or over ice.
• You can also freeze the juice in ice cube trays for easy portioning later.

Thank you for joining us on this journey through ***"The Diabetic Cookbook and Meal Plan for College Students: 110+ Diabetic Recipes for College Success."*** As you navigate the complexities of college life, managing diabetes can seem daunting, but we hope this book has provided you with the tools, recipes, and confidence to maintain a healthy and balanced lifestyle.

Throughout these pages, we have shared a diverse array of recipes designed to fit into your busy schedule, accommodate your budget, and satisfy your taste buds. From energizing breakfasts to hearty dinners and everything in between, our goal was to ensure that you have access to delicious, nutritious meals that help you manage your blood sugar levels effectively.

The meal plans and practical tips included are meant to simplify your daily routine, making it easier to plan, shop, and prepare meals that support your health. We understand the unique challenges that come with college life, and we've tailored our advice to help you make informed food choices whether you're cooking in your dorm, grabbing a quick bite between classes, or dining out with friends.

Living with diabetes in college is about more than just managing your diet; it's about creating a balanced lifestyle that supports both your academic and personal growth. By adopting the strategies and recipes in this book, you're taking important steps towards achieving your goals and ensuring that your health remains a priority.

Remember, the journey to a healthier you is a marathon, not a sprint. Be patient with yourself, and don't be afraid to experiment with new recipes and meal plans. Adjust and adapt as you learn what works best for you. Your college years are a time of discovery, and that includes finding out how to best manage your diabetes while enjoying all the experiences that come your way.

We hope this book has inspired you to take charge of your health and provided you with delicious recipes and practical advice to make your college life more enjoyable and successful. Here's to your continued health, happiness, and success both in college and beyond. Bon appétit and best wishes for a bright and healthy future!